the soothing touch
of
partner
massage
and
aromatherapy

brian green

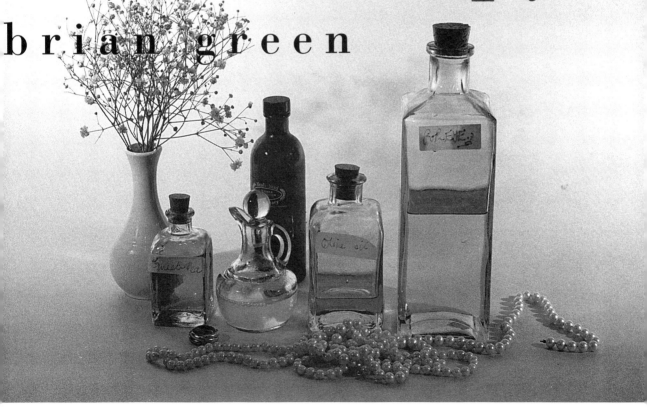

foulsham
LONDON • NEW YORK • TORONOTO • CAPE TOWN • SYDNEY

foulsham
Bennetts Close, Cippenham, Berkshire SL1 5AP

ISBN 0 - 572 - 01969 - 6
Copyright ©1995 Brian Green

All rights reserved

The Copyright Act (1956) prohibits (subject to
certain very limited exceptions) the making of
copies of any copyright work or of a substantial part
of such a work, including the making of copies by
photocopying or similar process. Written permission
to make a copy or copies must therefore normally be
obtained from the publisher in advance. It is
advisable also to consult the publisher if in any
doubt as to the legality of any copying which is to be
undertaken.

Printed in Great Britain by The Bath Press, Avon

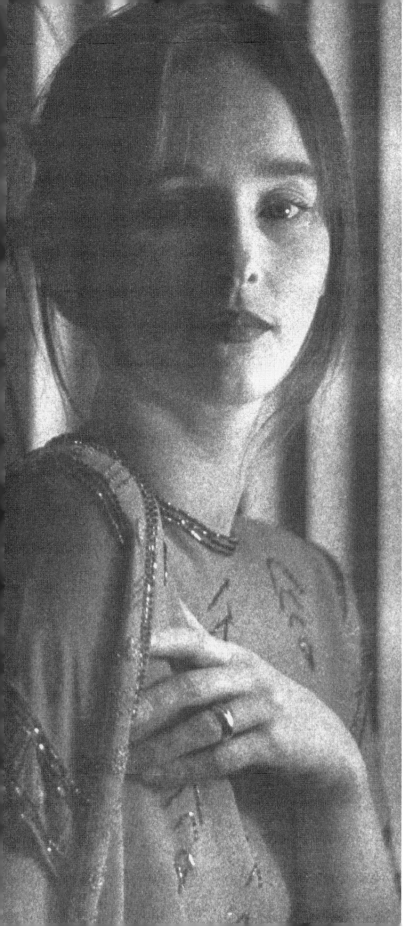

*Design
Photography
and Artwork
by
GreenInc &
Associates.*

*Make-up and Casting
by Amanda Lord*

acknowledgements

I would like to take this opportunity to thank the following people for their contribution towards preparing and producing the **PARTNER MASSAGE & AROMATHERAPY.**

CLARE PRESTON (aromatherapist) for the invaluable help and assistance she contributed towards the completion of this book.

AMANDA GREEN for the many hours of assistance given towards photography, make-up and production.

Models, PENNY LORD, ANNAMARIA WITHERS, ARIO ODUBORE (below), GEORGE TRIANT and IAN MILLER from the Urdang Academy of Ballet & Performing Arts.

ANTONIA AND TWINS, and LAURA HILLS.

HILARY CRAWFORD for her patience as 'Girl Friday'.

LYNDA TURNER (aromatherapist) for her invaluable assistance in the beginning.

EILEEN LLOYD (Editor) for her precise pen and judicious guidance.

And lastly, THE FLOWERS.

Brian Green

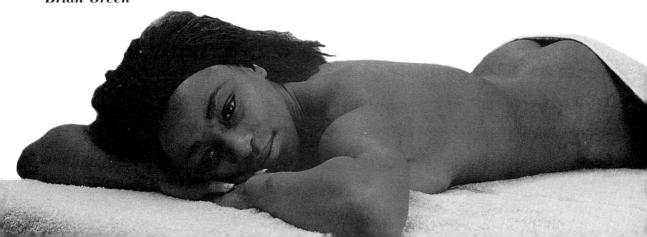

contents

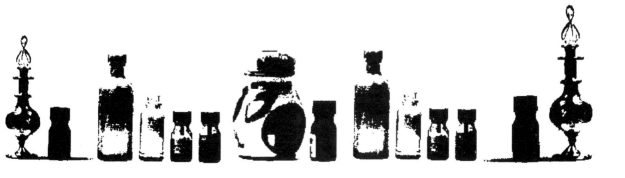

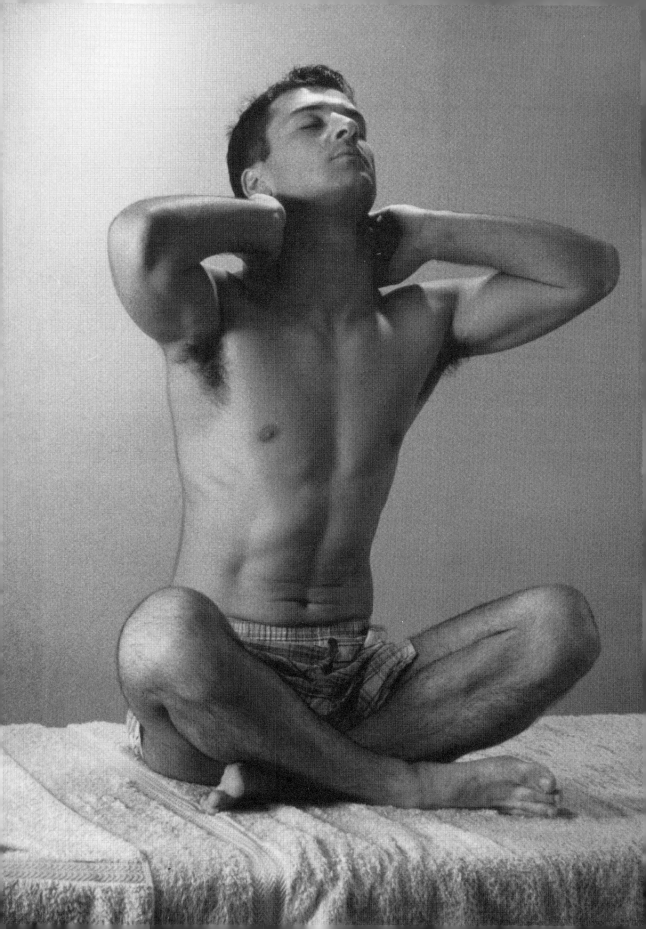

introduction

Stress lies in wait for us all and exerts tremendous pressure upon our daily lives. In this Hi-speed, Hi-tech era we need some form of relaxation to help us slow down and unwind.

Unfortunately for most of us the pace we live at has become a habit it is as though we have become brainwashed into fully accepting the demands that society makes on us. At the time of writing it was by chance that I happened to notice a daily newspaper heading saying: 'TEENAGERS "OLD BEFORE THEIR TIME"'. The article went on to say how a survey had revealed that life in the nineties was taking its toll on today's youngsters.

Stress hits us all regardless of our age or creed, and is always too ready to become our constant companion. However, not all of us are in a position to change or rearrange our lifestyle to eradicate stress. Most of us have responsibilities that we are unable to duck or put aside. This fact alone adds to our stress.

We can if we wish read various books on the subjects of diet, exercise, meditation and so on. Each offers us some method or technique that will supposedly enhance our lives.

'You are what you eat,' it is said, and the kind of food we eat is a root cause of many of our ailments. One way or another, our organism needs to defend itself. Massage can help keep the 'status quo' in your life, by promoting the correct functioning of the body.

Throughout this book you will find everything simple and non-technical as I have kept anatomical references to a bare minimum.

Many wince at the thought of their body being touched or manipulated by a total stranger. Most of us have been conditioned to expect that form of intimacy only from within a very close relationship. However, stroking someone's cat or dog in a gentle and caring way causes us no concern or embarrassment whatsoever. Why is this?

When we were children we were often 'rubbed' or 'stroked' by a caring parent when we had hurt ourselves.

Being touched was no problem to us then. It was only when we got older that we preferred not to be cuddled, touched or squeezed. We felt embarrassed, especially if you were a teenage boy.

I know for a fact that most developed males have initial difficulty in distinguishing between a 'sexual' or 'sensual' touch. A high percentage of females can appreciate a sensual touch without being sexually aroused, but the male enjoys being aroused and may even demand it. Fortunately, this 'sexual drive' can be educated into passiveness after several massages.

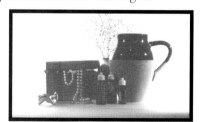

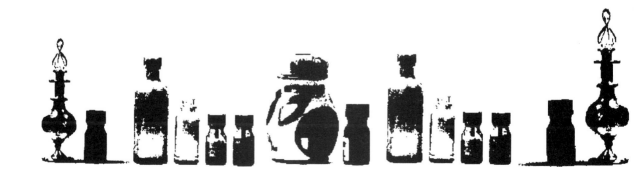

hazards

Many newspapers advertise either 'Massage' or 'Aromatherapy' in their classified advertisement columns. Most males would visit the former, and females the latter. Not many years ago the word 'aromatherapy' was not generally heard of.

Today there is an abundance of aromatherapists. This upsurge has brought with it a questionable standard of treatment together with many therapists needing therapy themselves.

Difficulty
Some therapists I have met have often shown difficulty in communicating their feelings and thoughts on a one-to-one basis and seem to have taken up massage to alleviate their own personal dilemmas.

A good practitioner in massage or aromatherapy is often difficult to find. To make matters worse, there are thousands of prostitutes who use the word 'massage' in place of the word 'sex' in

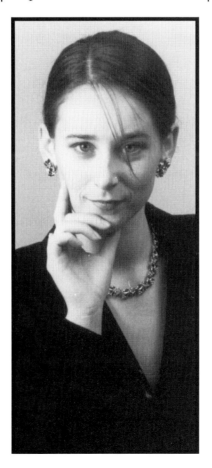

their advertising. From the male point of view there is no problem if you are looking for sex, but if you are ill and in need of genuine treatment there is nothing more embarrassing than being confronted by the word 'extras'. I should know.

In the early eighties I had been ill for some time and my doctor, who supported alternative medicine, suggested that I might try aromatherapy or massage to help alleviate the depression and anxiety that resulted after numerous minor operations. Not knowing there was any difference between aromatherapy and massage I searched the classified columns of my local newspaper under the heading of Health and Beauty. And there it was: 'A relaxing massage by qualified masseuse'. I rang the number and made an appointment for that evening.

Small room
I knocked on the door of a large private house and was let in by a woman in her fifties. She led me into a small room and asked me to undress and lie on the bed. She left the room closing the door behind her. Feeling nervous, I did what

I was told and sat on the bed and waited.

The room was lit by a dim light that was hidden behind a battered armchair. Heating was provided by an oil fire that smelt. I wanted to get out. My thoughts of escaping came to an abrupt end when the door suddenly opened.

Suspenders

Walking towards me came this woman in her late twenties. She was dressed in nothing other than black stockings, suspenders and bra.

I freaked out and spluttered something about my being in the 'Wrong place', 'Feeling ill', 'Had to go', 'Couldn't manage it', and 'Where's the door?' I left there feeling pretty shabby and embarrassed, even with some guilt of not being able to act the part of 'Macho Man'.

It didn't take me long to learn that you must ask what the fee is for a one-hour massage. If the voice at the other end informs you that they only do half-hour or 20-minute massages, you will know you aren't in for a straight massage. There are extras to be paid for. Be warned!

2 benefits of *regular massage*

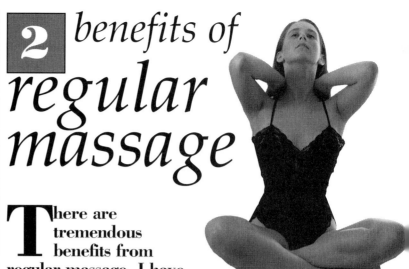

There are tremendous benefits from regular massage. I have always seen massage as an extension of yoga. Where yoga stretches the muscles and quietens the mind, massage quietens the mind while your muscles are relaxed and stretched for you. If you ever have the chance to massage a yoga pupil, you will immediately see the difference between a supple body and taught body.

Well-being

Massage assists oxygen back into tired and worn muscles. It also assists in cleansing and clearing the blood of toxic waste through the lymphatic system. Massage relaxes and quietens the mind while helping to induce sleep. It gives one a feeling of well-being. A regular massage is as beneficial as regular sleep.

3 *the basic techniques*

Massage techniques can differ in many ways, but basically they reduce down to four main groups: Effleurage, Friction, Tapotement and Petrisage.

These four main headings can then be divided further into numerous subheadings. But seeing that this book aims to get you off to a fairly quick start we will skip the many subdivisions and deal with the above four main movements.

As is the case with almost any technique, practice makes perfect. The saying 'hands on' is very apt when it comes to massage. The more 'hands on' you can experience the faster you will progress.

When you first begin to massage you will be frustrated time and time again at your clumsiness and a general feeling of being all 'fingers and thumbs'. Don't despair, as this is normal. And above all, don't listen to what your friends and acquaintances have to say about your efforts be they good or bad. Practise on friends at first, but don't forget that they are willing 'guinea-pigs' who have volunteered their body for you to practise on. They are not an authority on massage so aren't in any position to judge your efforts. You are your own judge and tutor.

Massage is similar to cooking. Once you understand what ingredients are required to create a certain dish you can then add your own personal touches to develop that certain something. So, learn the basics and add your personal flavour later. Massage is an artistic

expression by way of the senses and emotions.

Okay, let's get down to basics.

Effleurage (stroking)

Effleurage is probably the most commonly used stroke in massage. The word is derived from the French effleurer, 'to skim over'. It is a firm upwards stroking movement towards the heart using either one or both palms of the hand, followed by a gentle downwards stroke returning to the starting point.

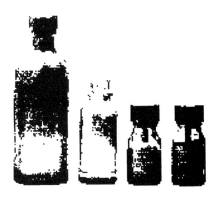

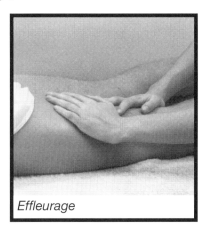
Effleurage

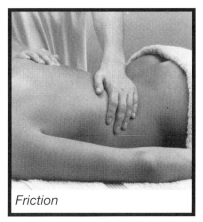
Friction

Friction (pressure)

Swiftly move the hands over the tissues skin, fat and muscles with a firm but not heavy pressure. Take care never to pinch the tissue because of obvious discomfort and risk of skin bruising.

Tapotement (hacking and clapping)

These are brief contact movements to an area. Your wrists must be very loose and relaxed or this can be an uncomfortable movement both for yourself and your partner. You can use the side of your hand, a loosely clenched fist or a concave hand.

Petrisage (kneading and wringing)

This action must be performed on relaxed muscles as these movements are deeper in their effect. Use the fingers and thumbs, heel of the hand or knuckles with a slow rhythmic action. Never perform this movement over any bony area.

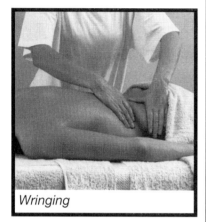
Wringing

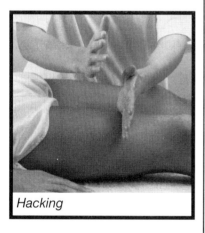
Hacking

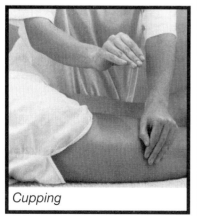
Cupping

4

getting started

First of all you will need to decide what medium you are going to massage with. Almond oil is one of the more popular base oils used, and can be purchased in almost any quality health shop. If you should have difficulty in obtaining almond oil then a good quality baby oil will suffice. Another popular medium is talcum powder.

Next you will need to decide where you are most likely to massage. This might well be on a bed, chair, table or the floor. If at some later date you should decide to invest in a professional couch then you will find such an item advertised in most popular health magazines. Often a strong kitchen table or dining room table is advocated for massaging on, but not many of us possess such items of furniture.

Two or three large bath towels or a soft blanket are next on the agenda. These will be needed for your client/friend to either lie on or be covered with. A pillow or soft cushion will also be needed as a head support.

Now let's get down to more detail.

Warmth
So often a masseur or masseuse will massage in an inadequately heated room with their client feeling cold but not wanting to complain. A vigorous massage can be hot work for the 'giver' but uncomfortably cold for the 'receiver'. Unless your partner is warm, he or she will almost certainly not feel relaxed or comfortable during massage no matter how hard you might try to please.

It should be remembered that a relaxed body requires outside assistance to maintain its temperature. With that in mind you should make sure that the room is warm and that you have either warm towels or a blanket to cover your friend or partner during the massage.

Peace and quiet

Another must for massage is quiet. There is nothing worse than being disturbed by a pet cat or dog scratching at the door, or when someone is thumping around in the next room. Even worse is someone unexpectedly entering the room. So, ensure that pets, children and neighbours are well out of the way. Finally, take the telephone off the hook.

I have a friend who religiously leaves a note asking not to be disturbed at the foot of the stairs before giving a massage.

Lighting and music

A dimmed or softly lit room together with gentle relaxing background music is of tremendous advantage in producing the right effect. There is a wide range of 'relaxing' music cassettes available from both record dealers and health shops.

If you are lucky enough to have a continuous play or twin cassette deck you will find massage to music so much easier than having to stop every 20 minutes or so to turn the cassette over.

As I am somewhat musically and hi-tech minded, I dubbed all my favourite massage tapes onto a VHS three-hour video cassette tape thereby leaving myself free to massage without the interruption of constantly changing or turning over tapes. Obviously I didn't want any flickering picture on the TV screen that might irritate my clients, so before dubbing the music onto the tape I recorded

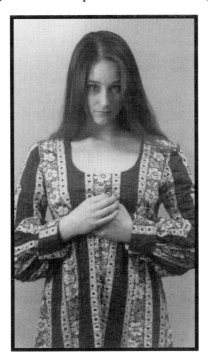

three hours of black screen with my video camera.

If you don't want to go to those lengths you can always dub your chosen music over any old video film you might have and just make sure that you turn off the brightness and contrast when massaging. Whatever you decide to do, remember the aim is to provide an uninterrupted massage.

Clothing

If you are massaging your partner, it doesn't matter too much what clothing you decide to wear as long as you feel comfortable. None at all if you should feel so inclined.

If you are giving an active massage you are bound to get pretty hot, so some sort of loose clothing is preferable. A pair of light-weight 'bottoms' and 'tee-shirt' are ideal clothing for most situations. I often wear an elasticised 'sweat-band' around my forehead when giving an energetic sports massage. This helps to prevent perspiration from getting into my eyes.

Hygiene

Personal hygiene is obviously very important when massaging, even if the recipient is your very

best friend. Body odour is one of the biggest put-offs you can offer. Remember, you are going to get very hot.

If you are a smoker, then scrub those hands and teeth. Even if you don't smoke or eat garlic, a mouthwash followed by an active gargle is advisable. Non-smokers are apt to pick up even the faintest whiff of tobacco. This should be done while your partner is preparing for his or her massage.

It goes without saying that a daily bath should be on the agenda. However, deodorants are not always a good thing because of the strong scent given off when you get hot. A tablespoon of a disinfectant such as Dettol added to your bath-water is a good hygienic habit to adopt.

Lastly, make sure your clothing is clean and fresh.

Fragrance

If you are the type of person who enjoys the fragrance of incense, joss sticks or essential oil burners, then go ahead – it can only enhance the massage.

In my experience an essential oil burner is by far the best form of fragrance dispenser. This usually comes in kit form and consists of a small round pot with a space left in the side where you place a night-light candle. On top of this is a container that you have previously filled with water plus a few drops of an essential oil. You light the candle, the water heats up, evaporates and carries the oil into the air. Again, these 'oil-burning' kits can be bought in most health

shops and popular market places.

I mention essential oils later in this book (see page 71). Aromatherapy is a subject in its own right, but it will suffice for me to say that a few drops of either lavender, orange or lemon in your oil-burner will produce the desired effect.

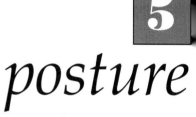

5

posture

Your posture is important. If you don't get it **right you will more than likely be needing a massage more than your partner.**

You should feel comfortable and at ease when you give a massage, otherwise your tension will be passed on to your friend. It does not take long to learn to relax the body when massaging. You will very soon find out that 'giving' a massage is as rewarding as 'receiving' one.

A bed can be very difficult to massage on because of its

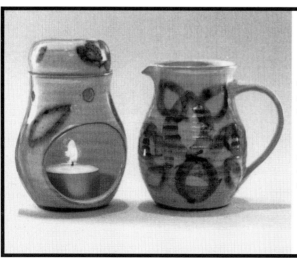

A typical inexpensive oil burning kit that can be found in most local health shops and stores

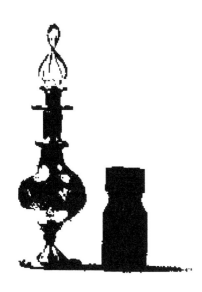

softness. The very nature of a mattress is to absorb the sleeper's weight, hence you usually both end up bouncing around like two corks on water. However, a bed does have its good points in that your partner is able to fall asleep during the massage and stay there afterwards.

You have a choice of either massaging on the floor, bed, table or professional couch.

If you are working on the floor, make sure that your knees are wide apart and you have some form of padding between you and the floor. Some people prefer to sit on one haunch with one knee at shoulder level. This is a good way to help keep balance. The floor is good in so far as you are able to use your full weight when it is needed but

this posture will more often than not make your back ache.

If you have a table or couch to work on, remember to keep your back straight and your legs wide apart. I mention the technique of 'rocking' and 'breathing' further on.

Though I find a table or professional couch much easier to use than the floor, I have friends who are most happy working at ground level. Again you must experiment to find out what suits you the best.

6
courtesy

I offer the following tips regarding courtesy and decorum as a guide should you be massaging someone you do not know too well. As I mentioned earlier, most of us are shy when it comes to exposing our bodies, even more so when it is to a comparative stranger.

A close friend of mine had just paid out a fairly large sum of money on a lengthy course on massage and the necessary equipment required to start up in business as a masseuse. This friend was apprehensive as to whether or not she would ever have any customers. I told her that she shouldn't worry as she was good at massage and would very soon recover her outlay. I went on to tell her that she would probably get more customers than I would on account of my being male. Needless to say, she very soon had more clients than she could cater for.

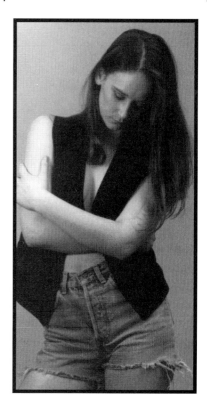

15

Because of the sexual barriers we have inherited it is harder by far for a male to set up in business as a masseur than it is for a woman to be a masseuse. Most western countries have the same outlook on massage, i.e. it is sexual. It is more common for a female to prefer to be massaged by a female than a male as her conditioning makes her feel safer in the presence of a female, whereas the male prefers to be massaged by a female.

Without going into any deep psychological analysis, it is generally accepted that the female feels initially uncomfortable about being massaged by a man. Bearing that in mind, let us continue.

Don't stand around while your friend or client undresses. Tell them that you are off to wash your hands while they get themselves ready. Explain clearly how they should lie and ask them to cover themselves with the full-size bath-towel that you have left neatly folded and provided for them. Be friendly but efficient. Dim the lights and switch on the soft music.

Embarrassment

Clients differ in what parts of their anatomy they would much prefer to hide. Some apologise for their large or more often than not cold feet. Some display embarrassment at being overweight. The most common anxiety is that their tummy is too large and that they really must lose weight. I once had a fragile seven stone anorexic ashamed that she was too fat and flabby.

We all have our ideal figure in mind, and would very much like to accomplish it. However, we are what we are and must accept things as they are. If we do not, then misery is our lot.

Most of our dislikes for our anatomy are a habit that began many years ago. Fortunately, others don't see us in the same light as we often see ourselves.

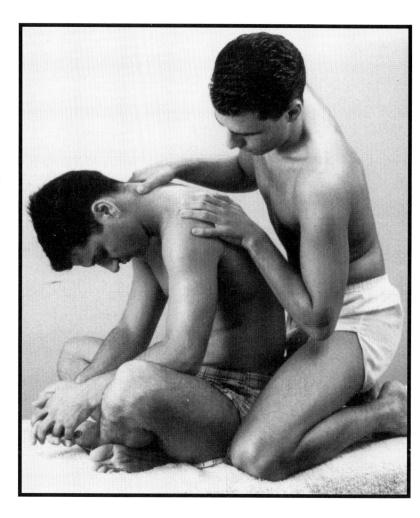

7

tips

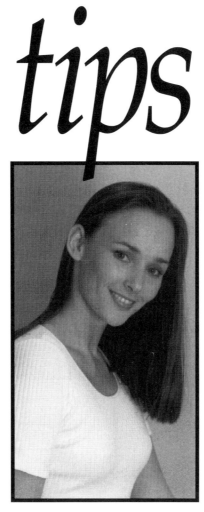

S ometimes the brain can get into a mess when it tries to assimilate more knowledge than it can cope with at one time. So I hope the following list of tips will alleviate this problem to some degree. Copy or photostat it and keep it handy while massaging in your early days.

A few do's to remember

Do keep your client's feet cosy, covered and warm.

Do keep the room warm during massage.

Do use warm oil when starting massage.

Do blow your nose if you feel you are going to sniff.

Do keep physical contact all through the massage.

Do often ask if your client is feeling okay.

Do support the back of the knee when lifting a leg.

Do offer the choice of a pillow to support the head.

Do encourage deep breathing.

Do keep a firm hold when lifting any limb or the head.

Do give words of encouragement when your client relaxes.

Do be firm and sure with your technique.

Do be gentle when massaging the stomach.

Do be aware of any varicose veins or rashes.

Do avoid hacking any bony areas.

Do avoid eye contact during massage.

Do request that your client removes his or her jewellery.

Do allow your client to wear his or her wedding ring if he or she wishes to do so.

Do keep a cheerful but formal attitude.

Do refuse massage if your client has just been drinking or eating heavily.

Do ask if your client is on her period.

Do request that your client informs you of any physical or psychological problems he or she might have.

Do remember to provide your client or friend with a glass of water or a refreshing drink when he or she awakes.

A few don'ts to remember

Don't forget to warm the oil before applying it to your client.

Don't forget to knock or

cough just before entering the room.

Don't stare at your client.

Don't apologise for your creaking joints.

Don't comment on any part of your client's body unless it is of a supportive nature.

Don't start by going on about your personal problems, I doubt your client will want to know.

Don't drink or eat in the room.

Don't break physical contact or leave the room once you have begun your massage.

Don't interrupt your client unless asked a direct question.

Don't sit on the side of the couch or table.

Don't apologise if you accidentally touch a sensitive spot.

Don't pour oil directly onto your client's body.

Don't leave any part of your client's body uncovered that you aren't immediately working on.

Don't breath or cough directly towards your client.

Don't bump into the table

or couch.

Don't sniff.

Don't have the music too loud.

Don't make sudden movements.

Don't pause or hesitate over your next movement.

Don't keep knocking over the massage oil.

Don't lean across your client to reach for something.

Don't lift the legs by the feet only.

Don't use hacking on any bone areas.

Don't make eye contact during massage.

Don't massage your client if he or she has been drinking or eating heavily.

Don't forget to provide a glass of water or refreshing drink after the massage.

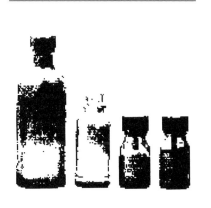

a guide to when massage is NOT desirable

1 In cases of fever.

2 Over or near a recent fracture.

3 Over varicose veins.

4 Over recent sore tissue.

5 Over dilated capillaries.

6 Over any unhealed or recently healed wounds.

7 Over metal pins or plates.

8 Over inflamed areas of any nature.

9 Over any septic area of the skin.

10 Over any unidentified pain or swelling.

11 In cases of any skin disease.

12 During late pregnancy.

13 In weak heart conditions.

14 In cases of high or low blood pressure.

15 In cases of lung disease.

16 Rheumatic or arthritic joints.

17 Very swollen limbs.

18 Swollen ankles due to causes other than long periods of standing.

19 Abdominal massage should not be given in cases of hernia or diarrhoea.

20 Where there is loss of skin sensation.

21 In cases of obesity due to hormone imbalance.

22 Epileptics.

23 Asthmatics.

24 Diabetics.

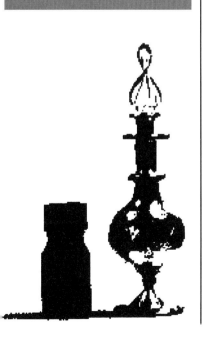

some 9 *comments*

1 If you have taken to a regular weekly massage, you may well find that by the fourth week you are able to feel relaxed and comfortable enough to drift in and out of sleep while being massaged. This is very pleasant to experience. You may also find yourself experiencing strong feelings, sometimes joyful, sometimes sad. Stay with it. You are getting closer to yourself.

2 If your friend or spouse has difficulty in sleeping at night, ask him or her to lie face downwards with their feet protruding over the end of the mattress. Make yourself comfortable at the foot of the bed and firmly grip their left foot with both hands while firmly stroking downwards with both thumbs into the sole of the foot. Begin at the heel and slowly work your way down towards the base of the toes making sure you massage the whole surface of the sole. Then gently change to the right foot and start again.

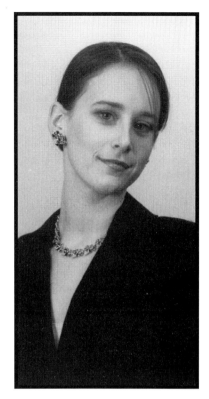

Five to ten minutes on each foot should be enough, depending upon the amount of stress your friend has been undergoing.

If you have the patience, try it. You'll find it works wonders. He or she should be asleep in no time.

3 In my experience most men are not very happy with the feel of oil on their body, especially on their face. It is usually best to leave their face untouched in massage. If you are able to massage without any base oil, so much the better. However, their dry skin may demand the use of either oil or talcum powder.

4 Long nails can be irritating and sometimes painful to the recipient. If you want to keep on the good side of your partner keep your nails reasonably short. There's nothing worse than being scraped or scratched when you are trying to relax.

5 Many of us are 'ticklish' in some areas of our body, mostly around the abdomen, thighs and feet. This is perfectly normal and takes getting used to. However, you'll be surprised to find that after only a few massages the tension will disappear from these areas.

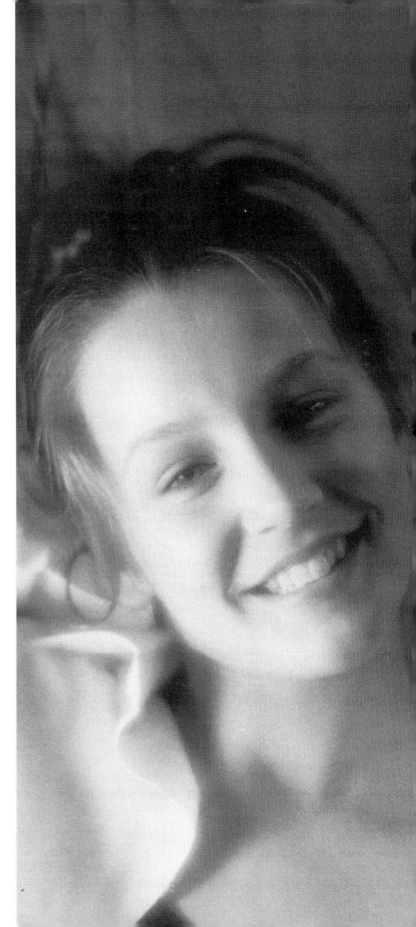

top to toe!

Whatever site you have chosen to work on, be it the floor, bed, couch or table, I suggest the following massage routine should be adopted until you feel confident enough to create your own personal routine:

1 Back and neck.
2 Buttocks.
3 Back of left leg and foot.
4 Back of right leg and foot.

Turn over.
5 Front of right leg.
6 Front of left leg.
7 Chest and abdomen.
8 Left arm and hand.
9 Right arm and hand.
10 Head.

Having previously requested that your friend or partner disrobe, he or she should now be lying face down and covered with a warm towel or soft blanket. Most people adopt a sunbathing position with their hands either side of their head. As long as they are comfortable it doesn't

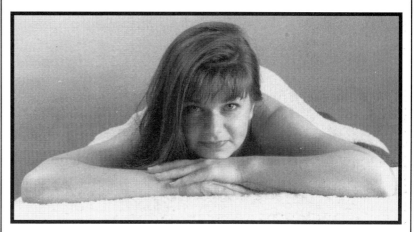

matter what position they choose.

It is preferable that your subject doesn't wear clothing, but if he or she is shy they should be allowed to wear, at the most, pants or briefs and bra.

Warm oil
With your subject lying on his or her front, fold down the towel to expose the back and buttocks. Pour a few drops of warm oil into the

palm of your hand and gently apply it to the exposed skin. Slowly work in the oil with both palms, not forgetting the sides.

The back
The back is the largest expanse the body has to offer, so some 20 minutes' work on this area would be normal.

He or she should now be lying in their most comfortable position. Most people choose a sunbathing position.

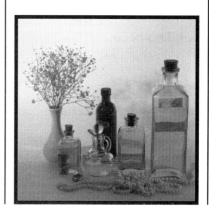

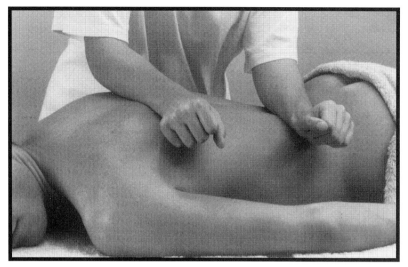

1 *With your partner lying comfortably face downwards, make a fist with both hands and place the inside of your forearms together in the centre of his or her back. Then, using your body weight, slowly and firmly pull your arms apart until both arms reach the neck and buttocks respectively.*
This first movement assists in stretching and relaxing the back and is pleasant to receive. Ensure that only your forearm muscle makes contact with your partner's back, otherwise you will have bone against bone discomfort for both parties.

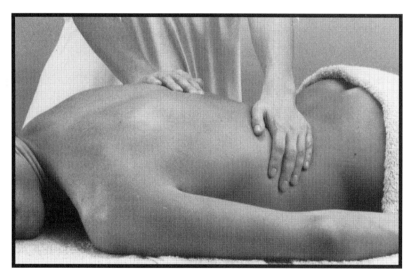

2 *Standing or kneeling to one side of your partner, apply firm and lively friction movements across the back. Begin at the buttocks and end at the shoulders. This is an invigorating movement that stimulates the blood vessels beneath the skin.*

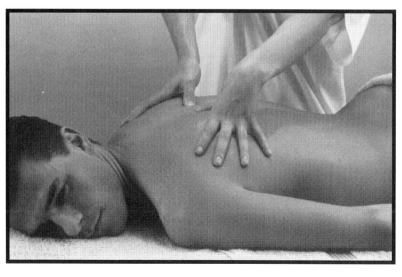

3 *Having placed both palms on the shoulders gently make small circles with the thumbs between and on the shoulder blades. More often than not you will discover small lumps beneath the skin. Gently massage these deposits. After a few treatments these lumps should break down and disappear. If your partner is undergoing stress this treatment will help relieve it.*

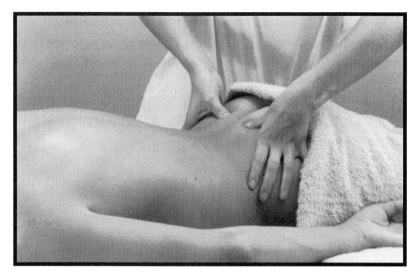

4 *Repeat the circular friction movement with the thumbs. But this time begin at the base of the spine and slowly work your way, one muscle at a time, up the two large back muscles situated either side of the backbone until you reach the shoulders.*

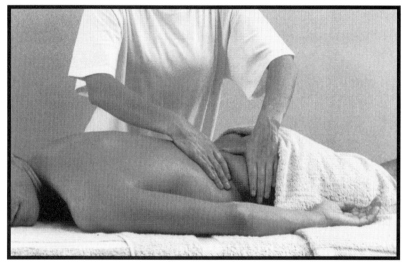

5 *Standing or kneeling to one side of your partner, massage the opposite side. With the palms of your hands, gently but firmly make passes from the hip to the armpit.*

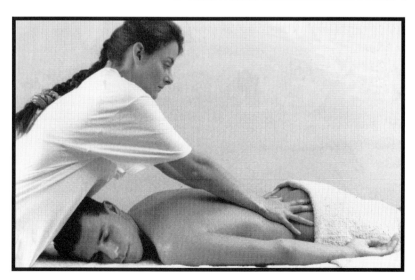

6 *Having positioned yourself at your partner's head, glide both palms down either side of the backbone from the shoulders to the buttocks. Then, with the fingertips gently caressing the skin, glide back up to the shoulders and repeat this movement several times. Because of the very nature of your position you can exert most of your body weight into your hands. This movement encourages the two large muscles positioned either side of the spine to relax.*

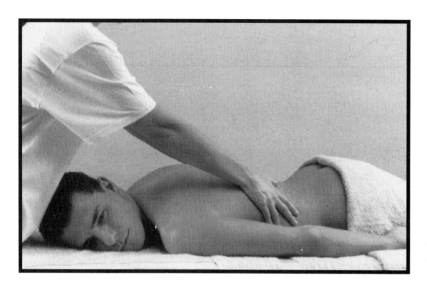

7 *Following on the movement from the previous photo gently and strokingly draw your hands slowly up to the shoulders to finish.*

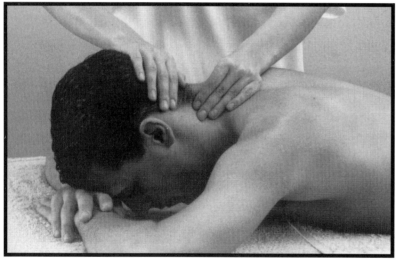

NECK AND SHOULDERS
8 *Having asked your partner to straighten his or her neck by placing their forehead on the backs of their hands, make gentle upward strokes from the base of the neck to just below the ears. If you are right-handed, this movement is best accomplished by placing your left hand on the back of the head while making a sort of sewing movement up the neck with your other hand.*

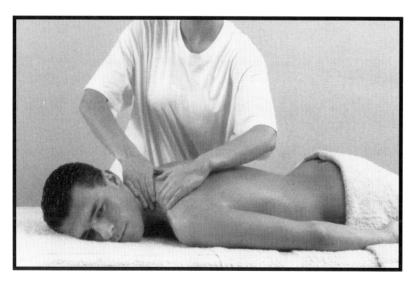

9 *Massage deeply into either side of the neck muscles and tops of shoulders.*

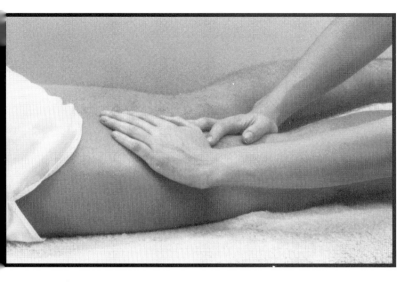

BACKS OF LEGS
10 Uncover the back of the first leg and sparingly apply massage oil to the full length of the leg. Position yourself at the foot of your partner and make gentle but firm upward strokes to the full length of the leg beginning at the base of the calf muscle and ending at the buttocks. Then gently slide your hands back down to the ankle and repeat several times. Do not apply weight to the backs of the knees.

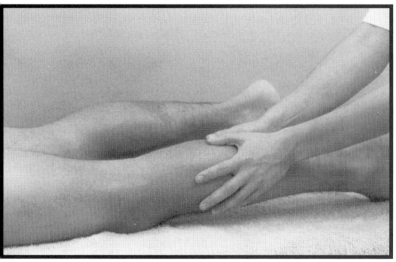

11 Massage the calf by gripping the leg with both palms just above the ankle and gently but firmly slide your hands up to just below the back of the knee.

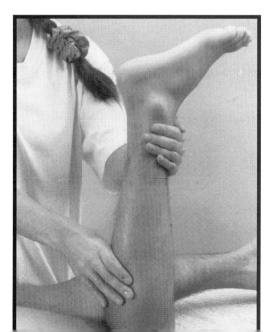

12 Raise your partner's leg to an angle of 90 degrees, and while firmly holding the ankle make strong downward strokes to the calf with the palm of your hand.

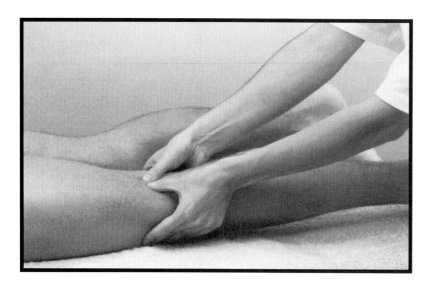

13 *Beginning at the base of the calf, make small circular movements with both thumbs up the centre of the entire leg. Skip over the back of the knee.*

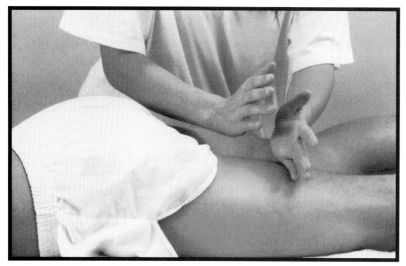

14 *With the outer edges of both palms, alternately make fast but light chopping strokes, from the buttock to the muscle areas of the leg. Chopping should not be used on the back of the knee or any bone area.*

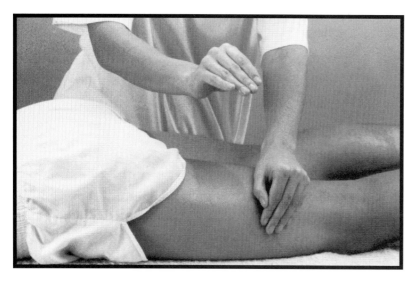

15 *Cup both hands and beginning at the buttock make firm and fast strikes to the muscle areas down the whole leg. This is a noisy movement but is good for toning the skin and relaxing the legs.*

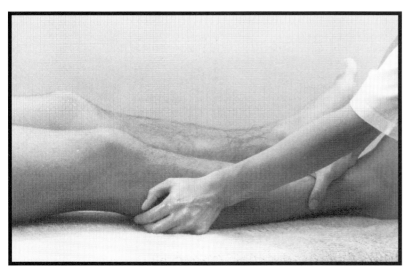

16 *With your partner lying on his or her back and having sparingly covered the front of the leg with oil, make firm stroking movements from the ankle to the groin. Remember to miss the knee-cap.*

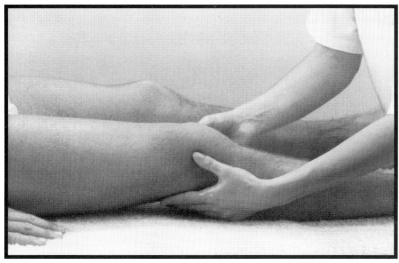

17 *While supporting the back of the knee and using both hands, very gently outline the knee-cap by making small circles with both thumbs. Do not apply any pressure to the knee-cap.*

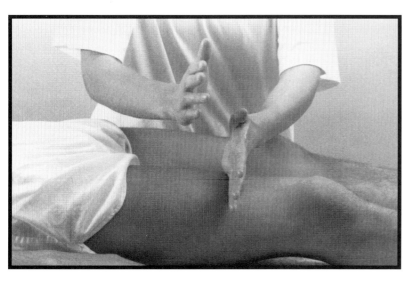

18 *Because most thigh muscles are tight, make fast but light chopping movements to the length of this muscle. Do not chop on any bone areas.*

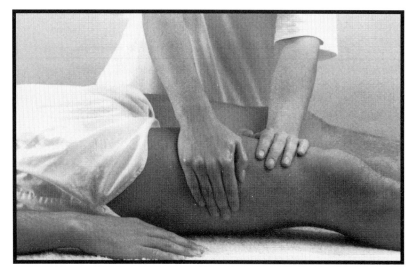

19 Make slow but firm friction movements across the full width of the thigh muscle, starting above the knee and finishing at the groin. This movement is achieved by firmly pushing away from yourself with one hand whilst pulling towards yourself with the other. This is a very strong movement that does wonders for tired legs, and it also feels great to receive.

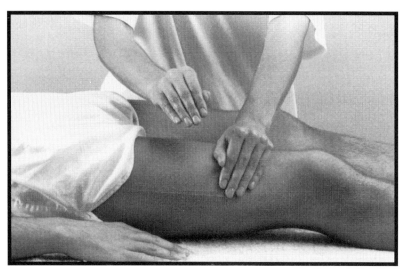

20 Repeat the same cupping movements that you used on the back of the thigh to the front of the thigh. Ensure that you get well into the inside thigh.

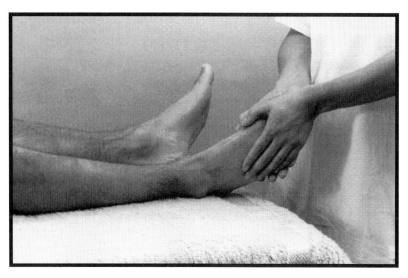

21 With your partner still lying on his or her back, begin massaging the feet. First, gently but firmly mould your hands into the shape of your partner's foot. Starting above the heel, pull towards the toes as if draining the foot into the toes.

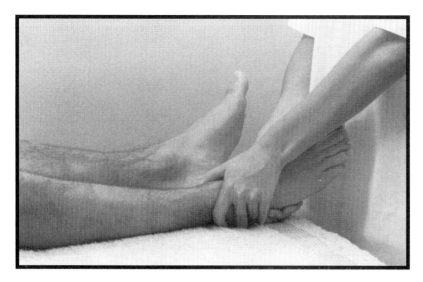

22 *Fit the heel of your hand into the contours of the foot and gently massage the sole, arches, sides and instep.*

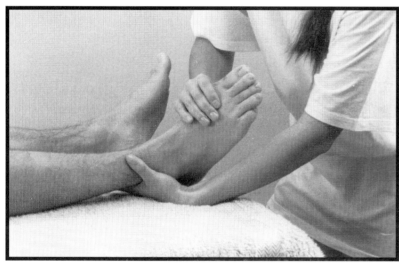

23 *While supporting the ankle with one hand, massage the sides and back of the heel with the other.*

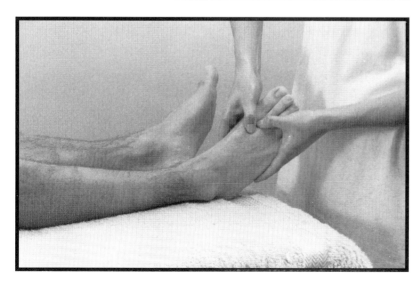

24 *Gently massage between the knuckles of the toes by making alternate short pulling movements with the thumbs.*

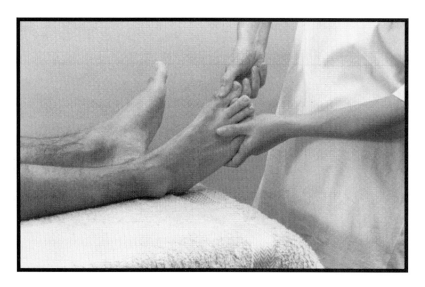

25 *With your thumb and forefinger, gently stretch each toe.*

Abdomen

26 *Leaning over your partner, place both hands either side of the torso. Make strong upward strokes beginning just above the hip bone and ending just below the armpits. This movement is extremely pleasant to receive and does wonders for the respiratory system.*

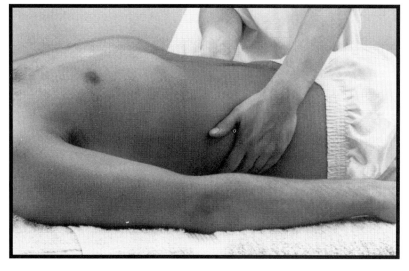

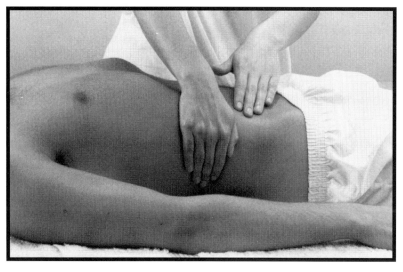

27 *Reach over to the far side of your partner and with alternate palms firmly pull towards you. Work your way from the waist up to the armpits.*

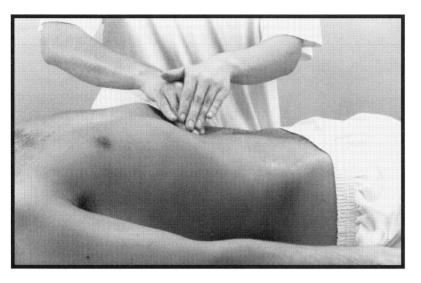

28 *Very gently make small circles with the fingertips in a slow clockwise direction around the abdomen. This can then be followed by placing the palms of both hands onto the abdomen and making large, light, slow circular strokes in a clockwise direction.*

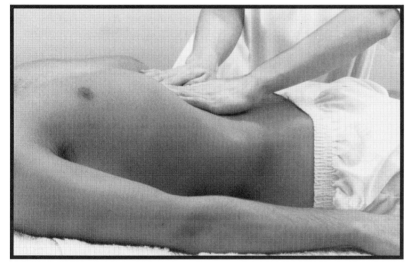

29 *Gently place both palms on the pubic bone and make slow gentle strokes upwards to the breastbone. This movement helps in relieving menstrual pains.*

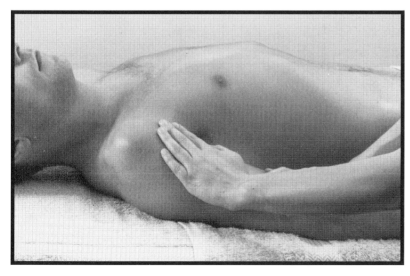

Arms

30 *Commence the arm massage by firmly stroking upwards from the back of the wrist to the shoulder joint.*

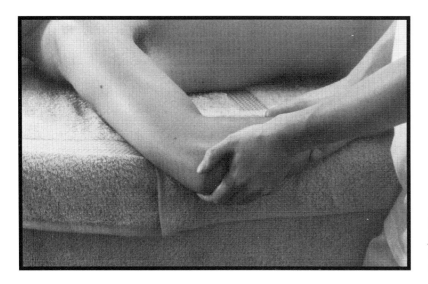

31 *Gently massage the elbow joint followed by firmly stroking up the inside of the upper arm from the elbow to the armpit.*

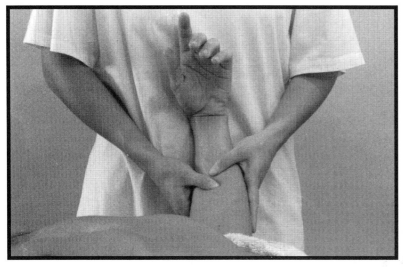

32 *While resting your partner's hand on your chest, apply gentle pressure with both thumbs to the wrist and then slowly slide both hands down towards the elbow.*

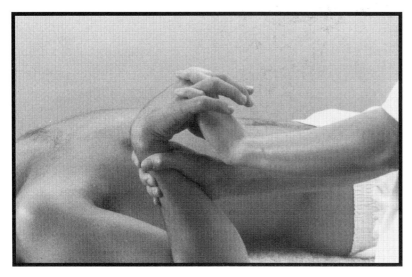

Hands

33 *While supporting your partner's wrist, entwine your fingers together and, with a slow stretching movement, pull both your fingers apart along the full length of your partner's fingers.*

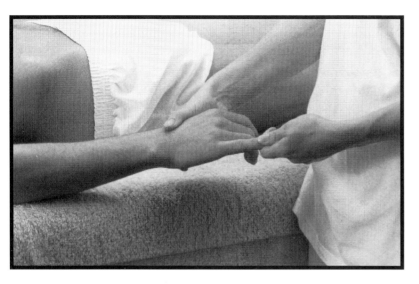

34 *Supporting your partner's wrist, firmly massage each individual finger joint with your thumb. Each finger should then be given a gentle tug to finish.*

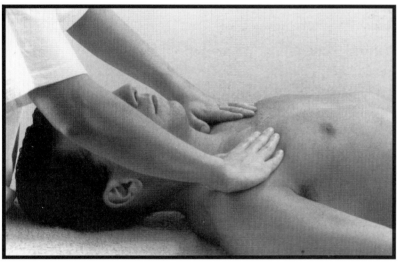

35 *Having positioned yourself at your partner's head, gently glide both palms from either side of the breastbone down to the pubic bone and then with fingertip pressure gently return via the sides of the body back to the breastbone.*

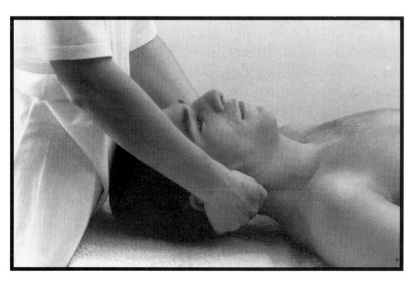

Neck and Head

36 *With upturned palms, reach under and between your partner's shoulder-blades and firmly pull your fingertips up and along the two large neck muscles. Stop, relax and repeat several times when you reach just behind the ears.*

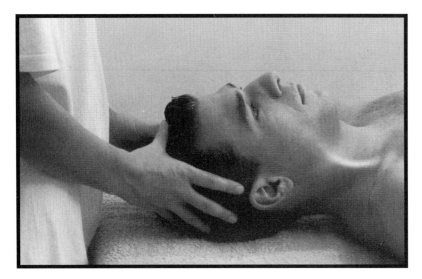

37 *With fingers spread wide apart, grasp your partner's head with both hands. As if washing your hair, make firm, slow and deliberate circles around the sides and top of the head with your thumbs and fingertips.*

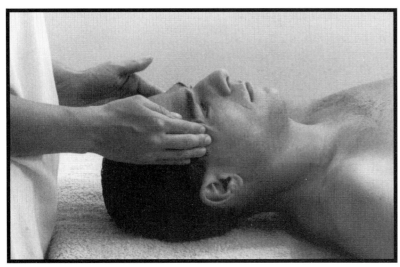

38 *Place your fingertips on your partner's temples and make small, gentle, clockwise circles. Occasionally, gently pull at the hair and tug on the ear lobes to help invoke a deep, relaxing sleep.*

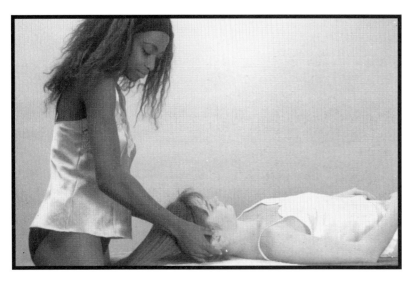

39 *Applying light pressure, place both hands at the base of the neck and make a long stretching movement up to and behind the ears.*

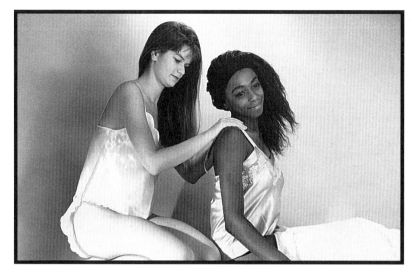

40 *Make a soothing stroking movement with the palm around the shoulders, finishing at the base of neck. Repeat this movement until you feel your partner relaxing.*

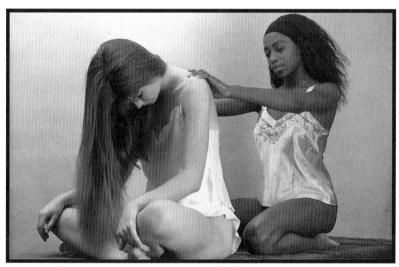

41 *Using small circular movements with your thumbs, work around the base of the neck and shoulders.*

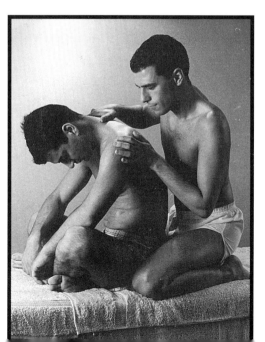

42 *Placing one hand on the shoulder, make light upward stroking (sewing) movements with the other hand from the base of the neck to just below the ears.*

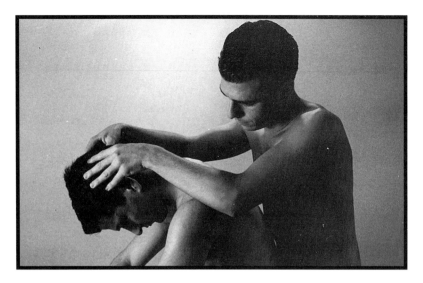

43 *Using all your fingers and thumbs, give a firm fingertip massage to the whole scalp. This would be similar to washing the hair.*

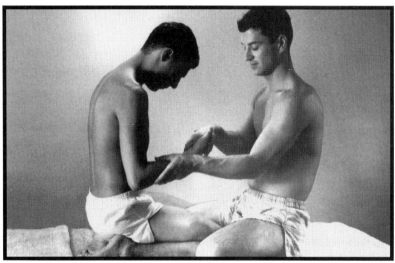

44 *Holding and supporting your partner's hand, make strong movements with the other hand by firmly sliding from the wrist to the elbow.*

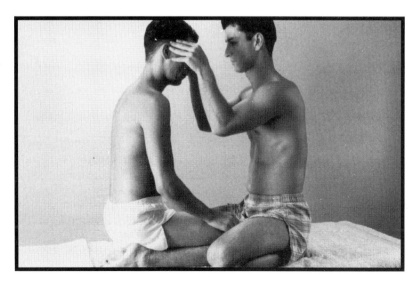

45 *First give light fingertip pressure and then make small circles around your partner's temples. Follow by placing your thumbs in the centre of the forehead and firmly sliding the thumbs out towards the temples. This is an excellent treatment for stress and headaches.*

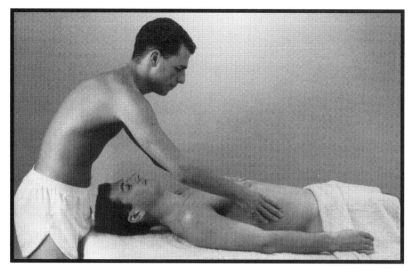

46 *Positioned at the head of your partner, make a strong downward movement starting from the breastbone and carry on through to the pubic bone. Then, sliding both palms outwards onto the hips, return with fingertip pressure back up the sides and around the shoulders and then glide the palms firmly down to the elbows. With fingertip pressure, slowly return back up the arms to the base of the neck.*

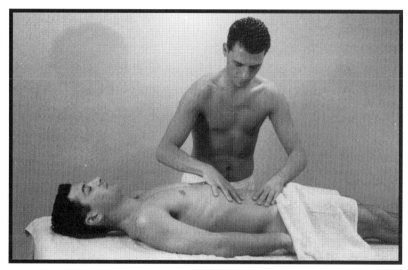

47 *Very gently place both palms on the stomach and make large circles with them around the abdomen in a clockwise direction. These circles should encompass the pubic bone and diaphragm.*

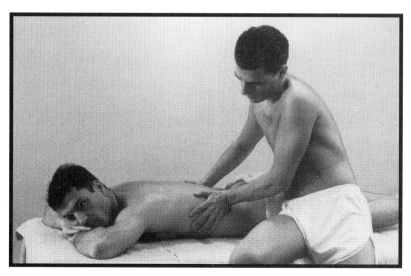

48 *Using the whole of both palms with the fingers separated as far as possible, apply pressure beginning at the buttocks and continuing up either side of the spine to the shoulder-blades. Return back down to the buttocks with a light fingertip pressure.*

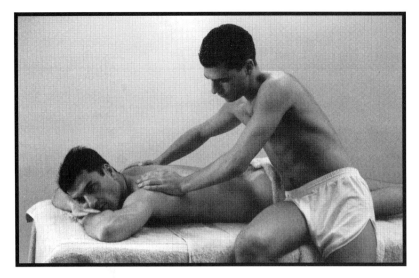

49 *See previous photo caption.*

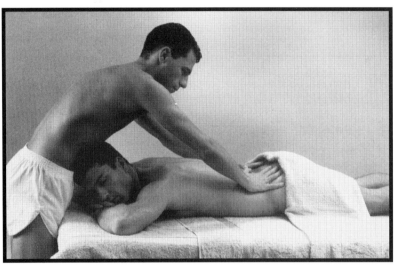

50 *Position yourself at your partner's head and, after placing both palms on the shoulders, make a strong, slow gliding movement down either side of the spine to the buttocks. Then slide both hands out to the hips and with fingertips only glide back up the sides, returning to the shoulders.*

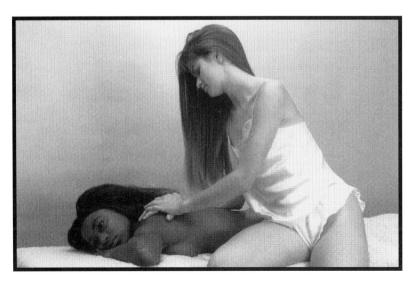

51 *With a double-handed stroking movement, start at the base of the back and slope upwards towards and around the shoulders. Sweep around the shoulder-blades and back down to the buttocks.*

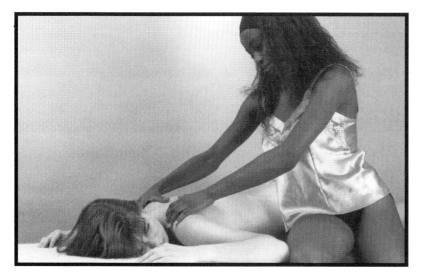

52 *Starting at the base of the neck and using circular thumb movements, work your way down either side of the spine. Then using a light caressing movement, return back up to the base of the neck.*

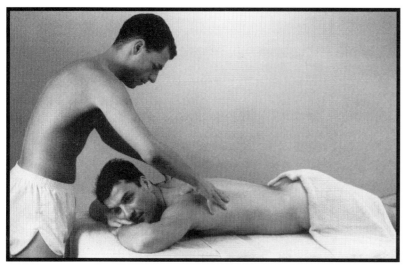

53 *With your fingers spread as wide as possible place both hands over the shoulder-blades and without breaking contact with the skin make strong, slow, firm circles in an outward direction.*

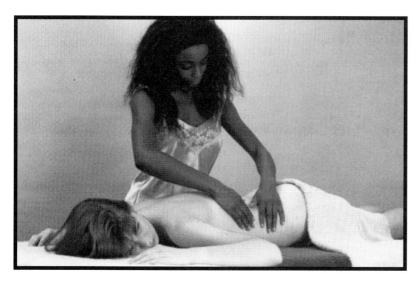

54 *Place both hands on one side of the waist, then making an action as if kneading dough lift the skin with alternate hands in an inwards direction.*

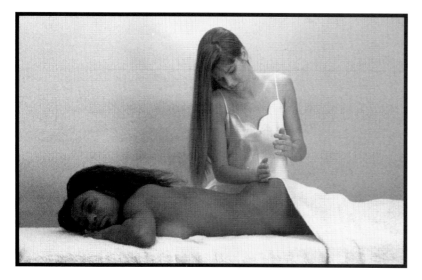

55 Using the little finger side of your hands, make a chopping action. This should not be painful and must only be used on fleshy and muscle areas.

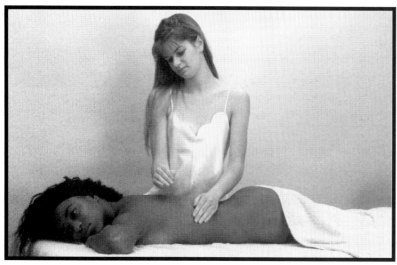

56 With cupped hands lightly pat the skin. Only use this movement on muscle areas as this can sometimes be painful to any bony areas.

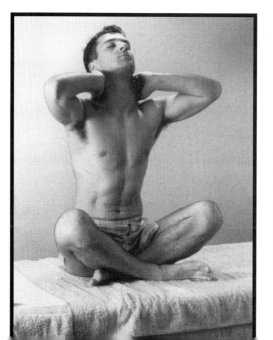

57 After the massage is over and your partner has rested, he or she should be encouraged to slowly sit up by turning onto one side first, so as not to cause strain, and then gently stretch the whole of their relaxed body.

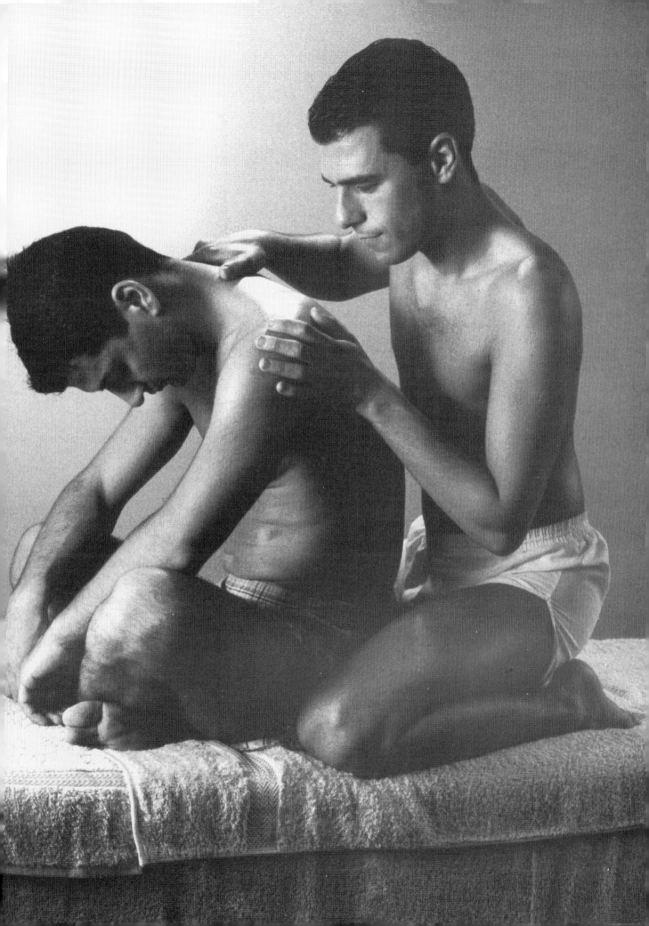

11 *facial massage*

The body, mind and soul each enjoy the attention given to it by its partner. Our face expresses all that we are and it too also needs and deserves the same gentle, soothing attention that the body receives.

A gentle but firm facial massage will soothe away exhaustion and anxiety and will leave you with a feeling of well-being together with providing a healthy glow to the complexion. Before starting your massage ask your partner whether they would like an oil or cream facial as some skin doesn't always take too kindly to one or the other, especially the strongly perfumed variety.

Supple hands

All you will need in the way of equipment is a towel, to place over your partner's chest, a headband if requested to avoid getting cream or oil into the hair-line, plus – and most important – a pair of gentle and supple hands. The last of these three is top of the list.

Before you begin your facial massage, place a warm damp cloth over the whole face to help encourage the opening and softening of the pores and induce the face muscles to relax. This towel should be left in place for a good three minutes before commencing with your massage.

By now any use of facial scrubs would have been discussed and included in your programme.

Your partner should now be lying on his or her back with head propped up by a firm cushion at the foot of the bed. You should be seated on a chair or stool at the top of your partner's head. Now remove the warm towel and begin the facial massage.

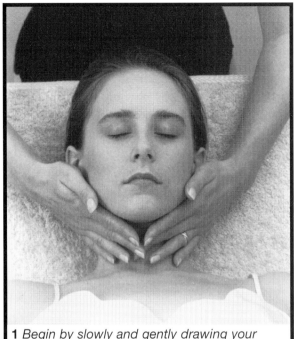

1 *Begin by slowly and gently drawing your palms and fingers up under the chin towards the ears, allowing your hands to mould into the contours of the face.*

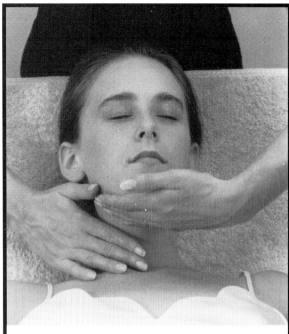

2 *Follow on the previous movement by working your way with alternate strokes under the jaw from one side across to the other.*

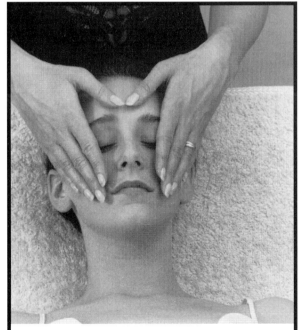

3 *Lightly place both palms over the whole face, then gently draw them outwards to the sides. Repeat.*

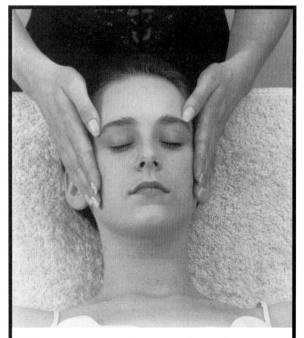

4 *Gently caressing the face relaxes the muscles and makes your partner feel comfortable and receptive.*

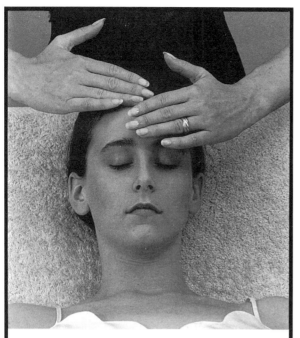

5 *Using alternate upward strokes from the brow to the hairline, gently massage the forehead.*

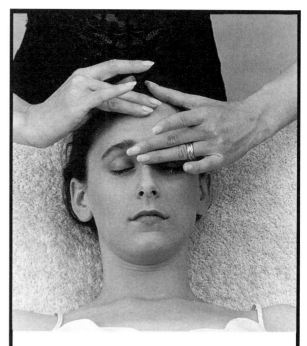

6 *Repeat the same procedure using only two fingers on alternate hands.*

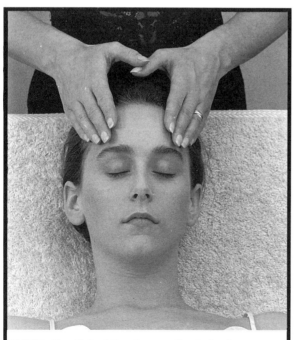

7 *With the flat of the fingers firmly in the centre of the forehead, gently pull both hands apart towards the temples.*

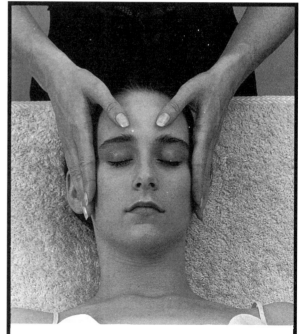

8 *While firmly holding the sides of the face with both palms gently stroke across the worry lines with your thumbs.*

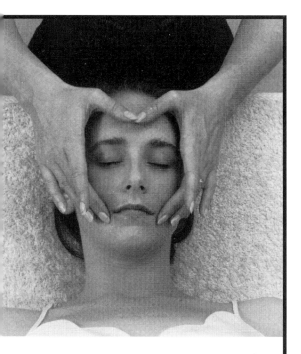

9 *Make light, upward circular movements at the corners of the mouth.*

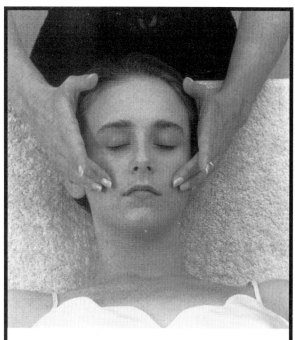

10 *Use light circular movements to manipulate the muscle along the cheekbone.*

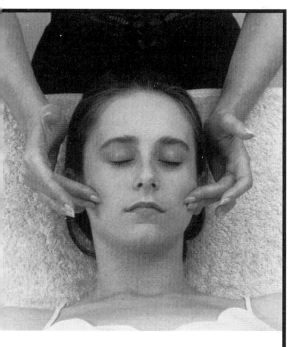

11 *Continue the manipulation along the cheek bone and finish close to the ear.*

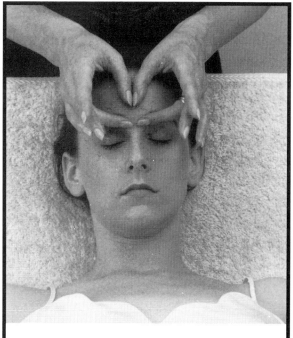

12 *With your middle fingers, very gently circle the eyes from the cheekbone to the eyebrow.*

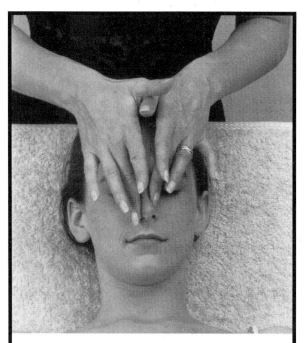

13 *Very gently make small circles up the full length of either side of the nose. Take care not to block the nostrils.*

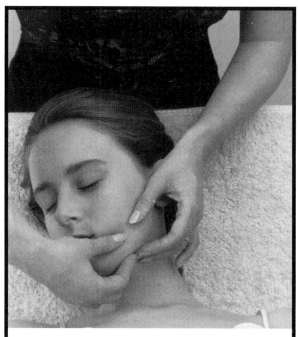

14 *Use alternate circling thumb strokes along the jaw-line.*

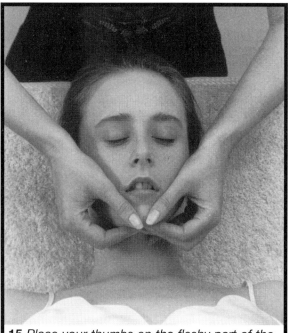

15 *Place your thumbs on the fleshy part of the chin and make circles with your thumbs. Then slide thumbs and forefingers along the jaw-line towards the ears.*

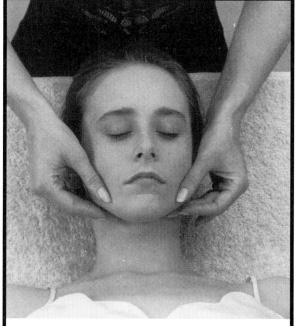

16 *Following on from the previous movement, slide your thumbs and forefingers along the jaw-line to the ears.*

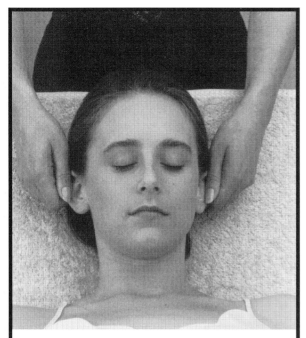

17 *Sliding your thumbs into the crevices, massage the whole of the inside and outside of the ears.*

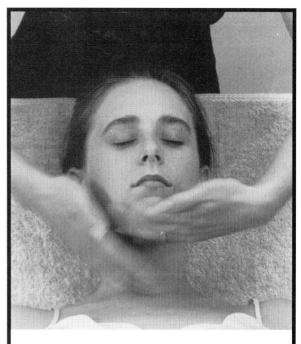

18 *Gently make light, alternate slaps to the underside of the chin.*

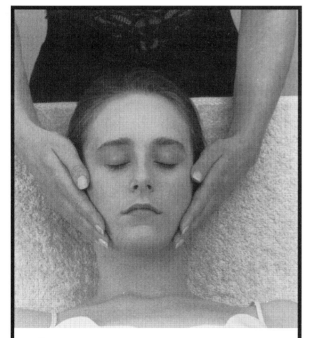

19 *Gently stroke and soothe the face with both palms.*

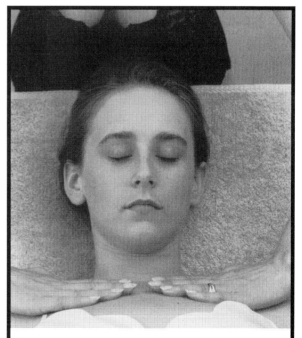

20 *To finish place your fingers on the breastbone and gently pull them apart until both palms are resting on the shoulders.*

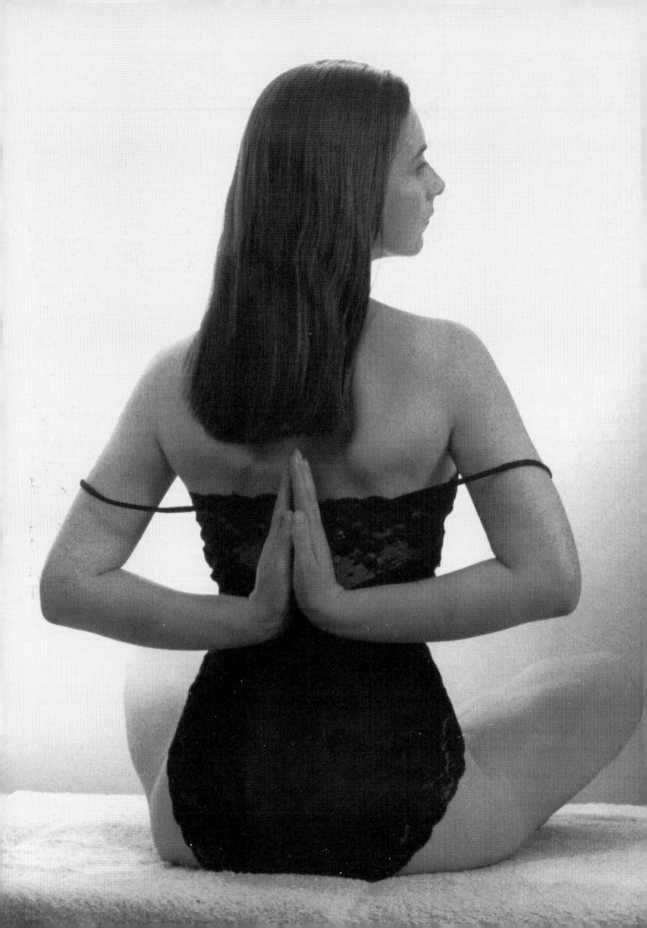

12 self massage

Some of us choose to live alone while others have had no choice in the matter. Old and young alike, we all need to care for ourselves in every possible way. It is much harder for the 'alone' person to receive the touch and care that he or she deserves.

There is a difference between being lonely and being alone, which does not necessarily entail feeling lonely. Possibly you are interested in becoming more alive, and are searching for something extra in life. To be sensitive to your body and how it functions contributes towards self-awareness. Maybe you have previously been involved in a sport, athletics, dance or yoga at some time in your life. Without dwelling too much on the esoteric side of things let's take a look at the benefits of self-massage.

Although it is very pleasurable and sensual to be massaged by another, it can also be very beneficial and pleasurable to be massaged by yourself. Obviously you will have to create your own environment as directed earlier in this book, with the right lighting, warmth, soft music, oil and a fragrance.

Self-massage can either be administered on the floor, chair or bed. Most popular is the bed. For the sake of convenience let us imagine you have chosen the bed.

First you must have adequate support for your back and neck, so I advise two or three pillows should be placed behind your head and shoulders. Personally I have found it very difficult to find a firm feather pillow, so you might have to resort to using the sponge-filled pillows that are on offer. However, a firm and comfortable foundation is required for your shoulders, neck and head. A folded blanket might well be successfully exploited.

With self-massage you will instinctively feel and manipulate the areas of your body that need attention and healing. If you are at one with yourself a self-massage can be more revealingly sensual and pleasurable than the touch of another. However, it might take a few attempts to get it right.

So, now that you are relaxed and quiet in your own environment let us begin.

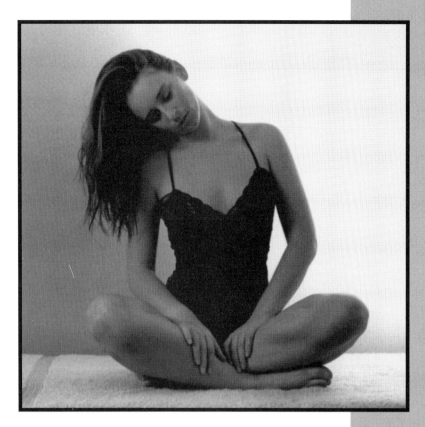

Sitting with your back straight, roll your head several times slowly from one shoulder to the other keeping your chin as close as possible to your chest.

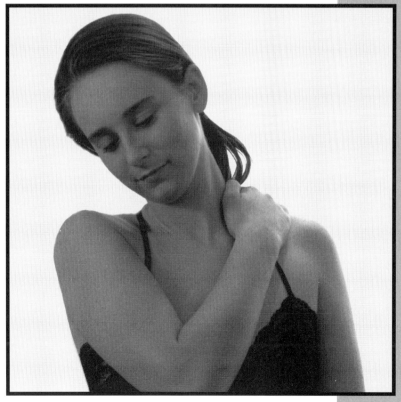

With your head tilted to one side, firmly massage the base of the neck with your fingertips. Repeat with head tilted the other way.

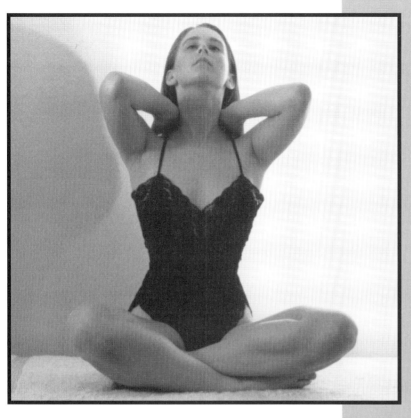

With both hands and fingertips positioned at the nape of the neck, firmly and slowly pull forward so as to stretch the shoulders.

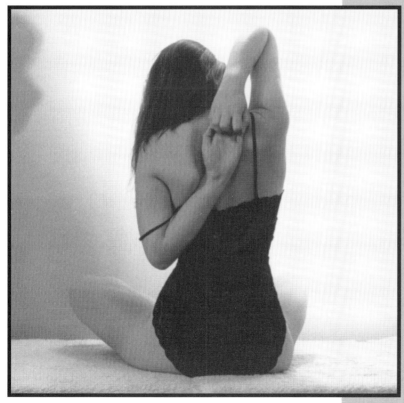

Position your hands as in the above picture and with your head as upright as possible hold this position for 30 seconds. And then change hands, sides and repeat.

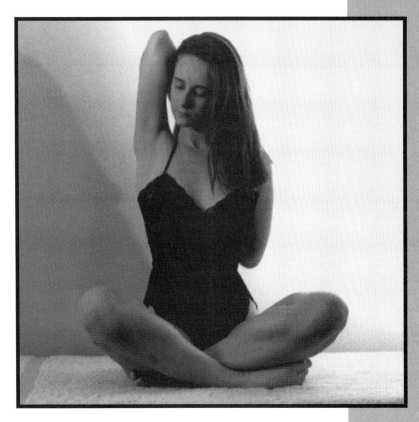

When you are feeling comfortable with the previous position gently pull apart your clasped fingers. Any student of Hatha Yoga will immediately recognise these positions and will understand the benefit they give.

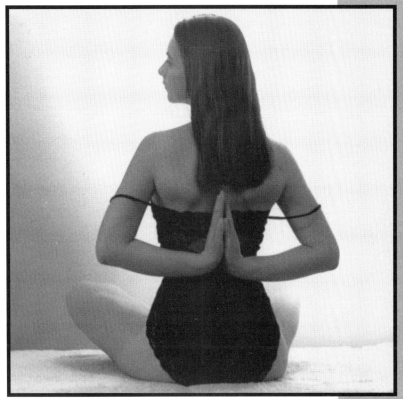

With both hands behind your straight back, try to force your palms together. It may take you a few attempts to do this movement correctly.

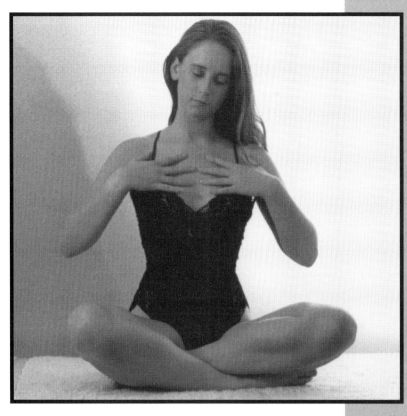

Position your fingertips between your upper ribs. Press hard and slowly pull both hands apart until they reach your armpits.

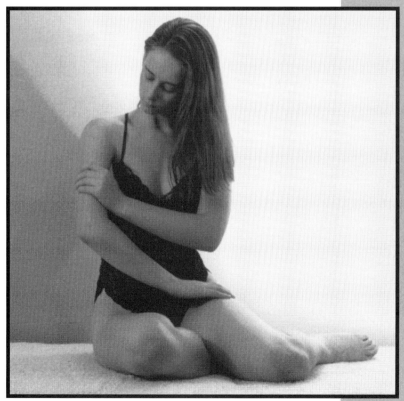

Gripping the wrist, firmly glide your hand up to the shoulder several times. Change arms and repeat.

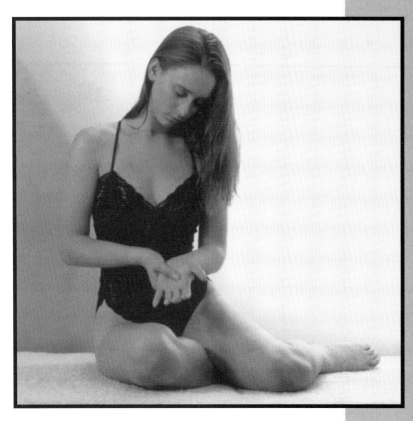

Make several large, strong circles around the palm of the hand in a clockwise direction. Repeat with the other hand.

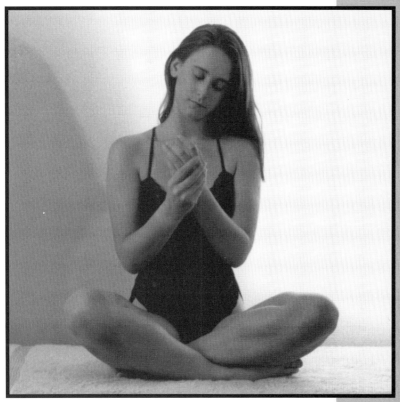

Press your thumb firmly into the centre of the palm and make strong strokes towards each finger. Pay particular attention to adding even more pressure when reaching the first joint of each finger.

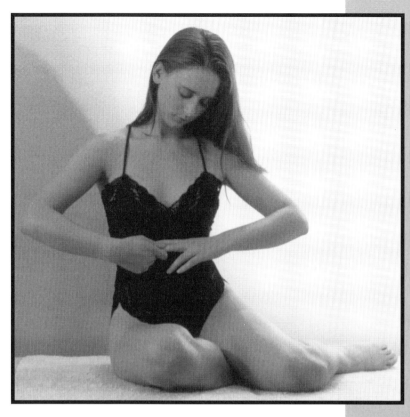

With your thumb, massage each finger joint, followed by gently stretching each finger.

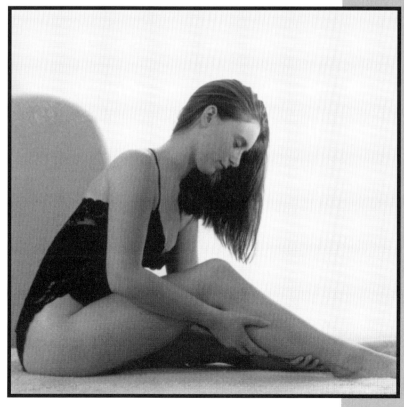

Bend your knee upwards and with alternate hands stroke the calf from the ankle to the back of the knee.

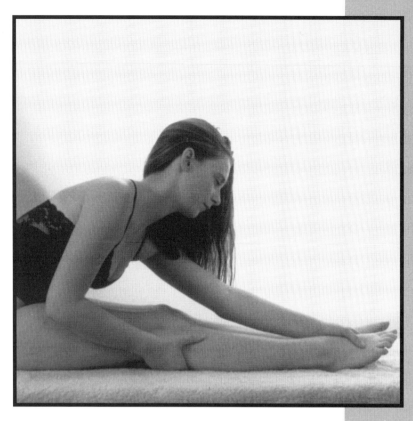

Starting at the foot, make long stroking movements up the inside of the calf to the knee.

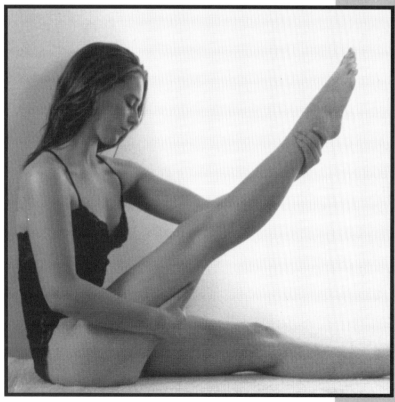

While supporting your leg by either the calf or the ankle, massage the back of the thigh from the buttock to the back of the knee with slow, strong strokes.

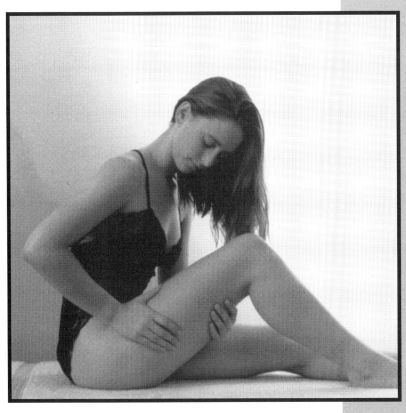

Using strong hands, grip the thigh and massage slowly and firmly up towards the back of the knee.

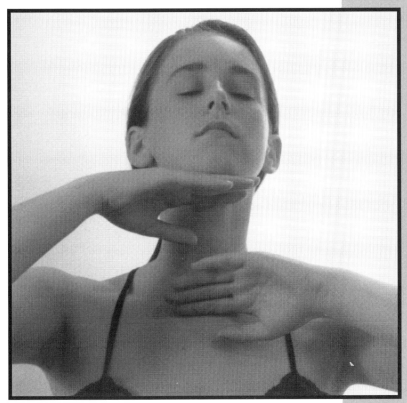

Make fast alternate back-of-hand stroking movements from the throat to the chin.

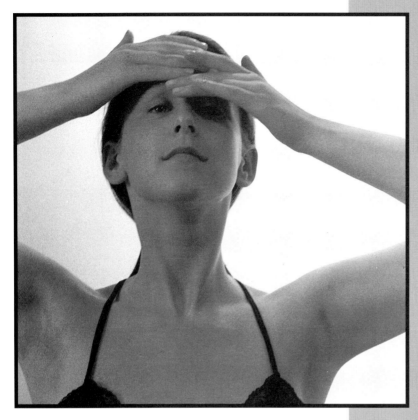

With strong fingertip pressure, make upward strokes from the brow to the hairline.

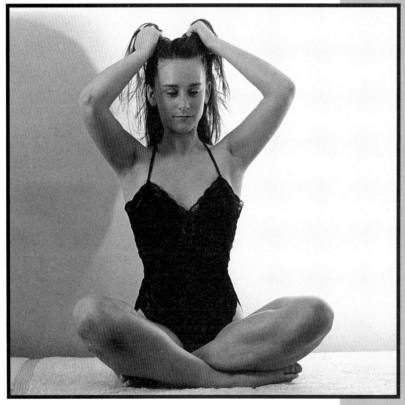

Gripping your hair close to the roots, gently pull firmly upwards. Repeat this procedure across the whole scalp.

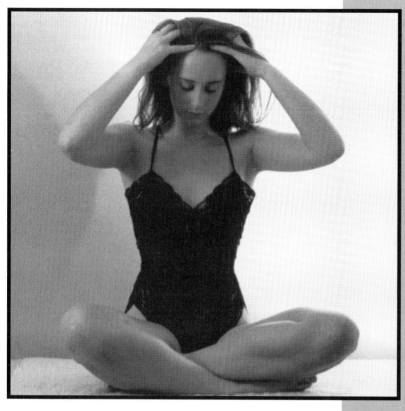

With your fingers and thumbs, massage the scalp as if washing your hair. Work from the hairline to the back of the head.

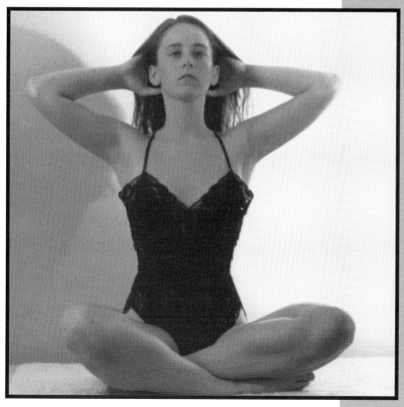

Continue this massaging movement from the base of the scalp to behind the ears.

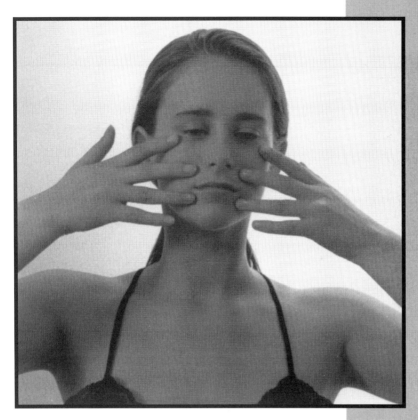

Lightly rotate the pads of your fingertips while slowly moving them across the face and back towards the ears.

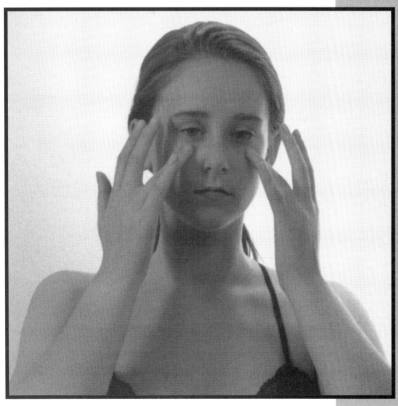

Using your fingertips, lightly stroke from nose to ears across the cheekbones.

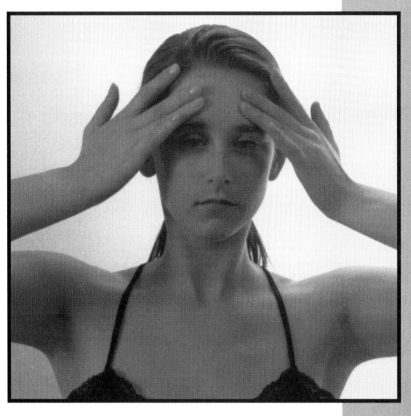

Starting at the centre of the forehead, press your fingertips firmly into your brow and slowly pull your hands apart until you reach both temples.

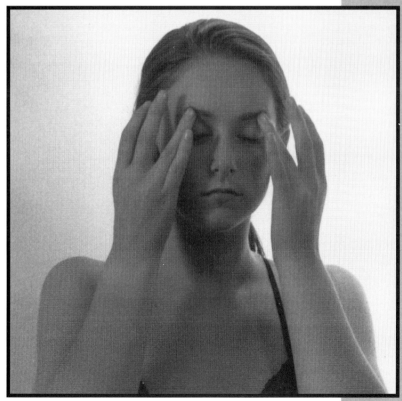

Using one finger-pad from each hand, make a very strong movement from the centre of the brow to the temples.

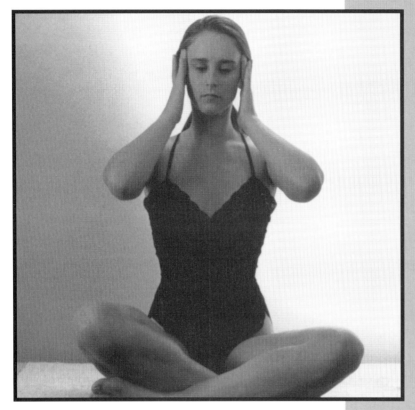

Using two or three fingers, apply gentle pressure to the temples and make small circles in any direction.

Having finished the above movements, lie on your back with your hands positioned on your stomach. While taking several deep breaths, allow your muscles and body to relax. If you should happen to practise any meditation techniques, now is the time to do them.

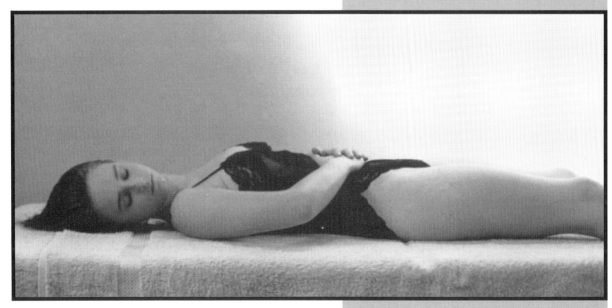

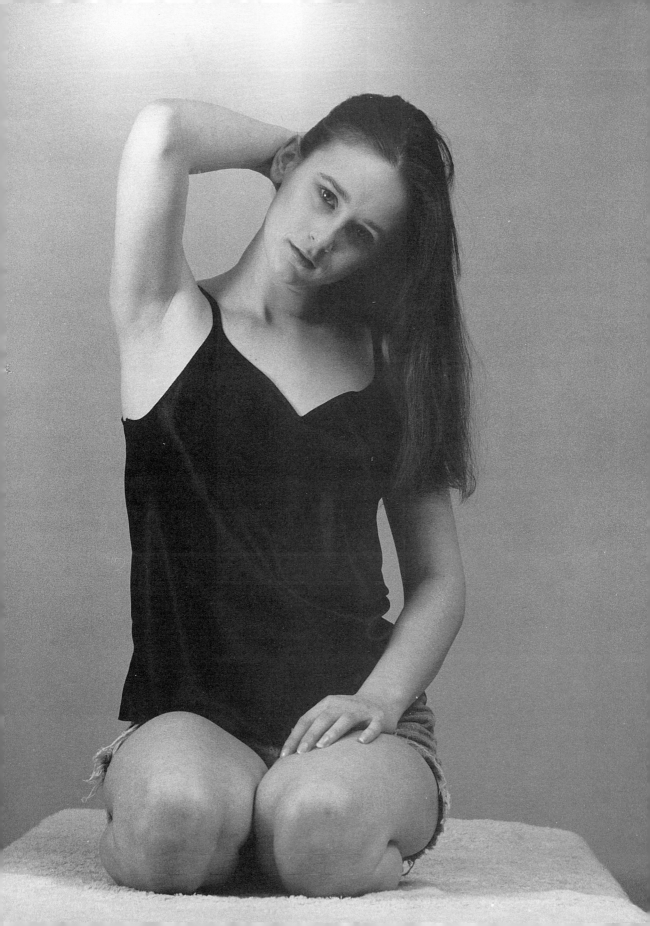

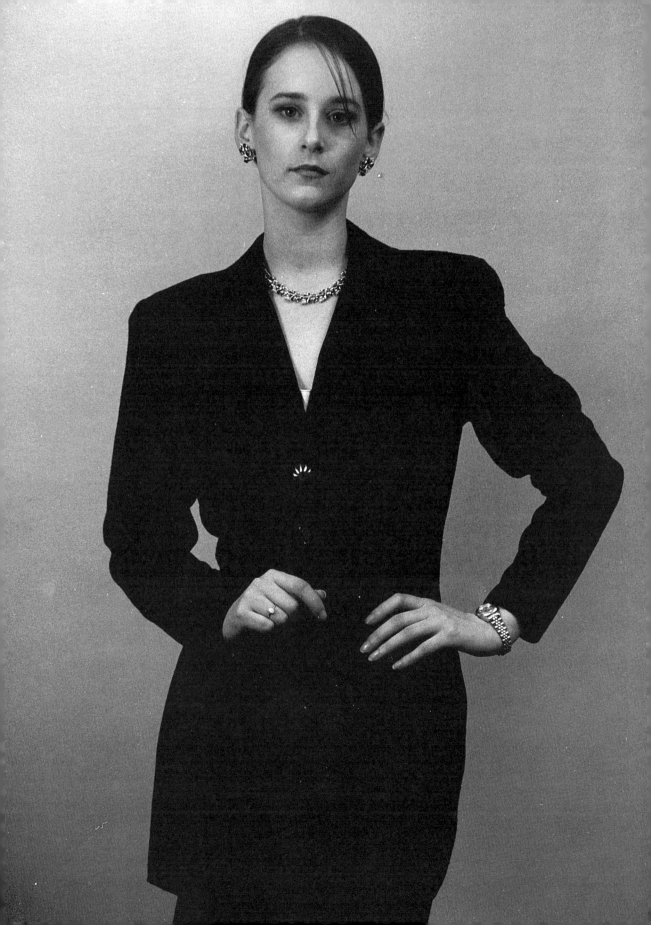

13

aromatherapy

Aromatherapy is seen by most men as a woman's 'thing'. Men tend to lean towards the feeling that sweet flowery fragrances are for the ladies and most definitely a 'no-go' area for them. However, they will splash on some after-shave when the mood takes them. This usually coincides with a party or some function where females will be present.

I clearly remember as a young man my splashing on lashings of my father's after-shave before setting off to meet my date. The male feels he will get his girl if he smells right. As he gets older 'smelling right' doesn't seem to matter so much. This blinkered attitude has left

aromatherapy firmly in the lap of the female. The male tends towards the bitter things in life leaving the female with the sweeter things. It is natural for the male to treat his female partner to chocolates, scent and flowers, whereas the male prefers physical rather than sensual gifts.

I have written the above in order to prepare the female reader for the let down she will more than likely receive when she confronts her male with a 10 ml bottle of pure lavender essence. He would much prefer to crash out on the settee with a six-pack of lager, an hour on his

computer or maybe a jog through the park rather than suffer the pangs of having to lay still for an hour whilst being smothered with sweet smelling sticky oil. Yes, I agree, not all men are like that. But, in my experience, most are.

So, ladies, if you would like to introduce your male to the more delicate and subtle side of life go steady on the base oil and even steadier on the essence.

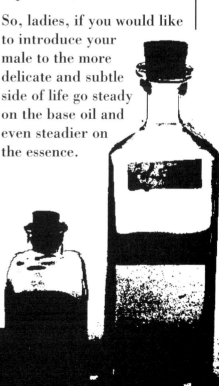

Hands on

I mentioned earlier that an aromatherapy course is by far the best way to learn the art of blending, mixing and applying oils. A book I specially recommend is *The Complete Book of Family Aromatherapy*, by Joan Radford (Foulsham 1993). Books are fine but they do not provide the much needed hands-on experience that is required. An experienced tutor of aromatherapy, however, can guide and assist you in the areas that the 'manual' or written word can't.

Expensive

Unfortunately there are pitfalls that you should be aware of before parting with any of your hard earned cash. Aromatherapy and massage courses are more often than not very expensive and need to be looked at carefully and individually before

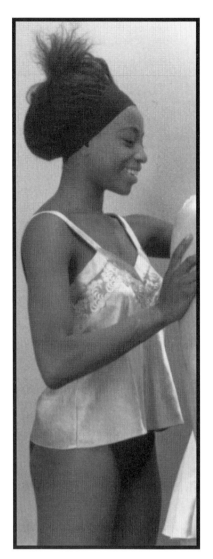

considering any enrolment. Many courses offer the promise of a diploma if you pass their examination criteria.

Anyone can offer a diploma in part exchange for cash as the law stands today. I could advertise 'The Brian Green School of Standing on One Leg for Two Hours' diploma, and would be well within my rights.

Bona fide

The point I am making is that you must ensure that the course you enrol on is bona fide inasmuch that it is nationally recognised and accepted in society's professional areas.

I can personally name many students of aromatherapy who have paid out hard earned cash only to discover that their diploma was not officially recognised. A letter or telephone call to the London based International Federation of Aromatherapists would not go amiss in establishing the credibility of your tutor. This action might well save you a lot of frustration and disappointment later.

Obviously the aforementioned text is directed towards persons who are interested in taking up aromatherapy and massage as a full-time occupation. For those of us who just wish to add another dimension to our lives, read on.

Unfortunate

It is unfortunate that many of us don't realise and fully understand the worth of aromatherapy and massage. Some ten years ago I was undergoing regular surgery to remove cancerous polyps that would not go away. This repeated and much feared surgery began to take its toll. I became depressed and ill in heart and mind. Life was becoming a burden.

In desperation I tried various holistic methods offered to pull the mind and soul together – I was determined to overcome this situation.

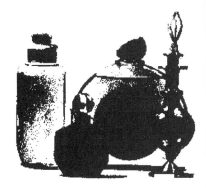

After many months of exhaustive searching and experiencing the innumerable techniques there are on offer for healing the body, I stumbled upon massage and aromatherapy.

From that day, my health took a turn for the better and I have never looked back.

My weekly health routine consisted of swimming, massage and yoga. Massage helped my body overcome the stress that regular surgery had placed upon it. My strength and energy to fight back at long last returned.

Incense

I mentioned earlier that aromatherapy is not a new thing to society. If what historians have claimed is true it is amazing to think that as long ago as 3000 BC Egyptian priests and priestesses were burning resins of frankincense. Later, the Romans used to burn incense in their homes, and took hot scented baths and regular massage.

To think that in those days you would have been regarded as an elderly person at 30 years of age!

Black Death

During the time of the Black Death herbalists prepared such herbs as rosemary and peppermint to help ward off the plague. It is also interesting to read that in 1937 a Frenchman, René Gatefoss, coined the word 'aromatherapy'. Apparently, while in his laboratory he accidentally burnt his hand. Immediately he plunged his arm into a nearby bowl containing essential oil of lavender. To his amazement the pain quickly subsided, and the burn subsequently healed without leaving a scar.

Research

Being a chemist he soon realised that properties within the essence of lavender were healing and antiseptic, which lead him to investigate further the qualities that flowers and herbs contained. Among others, the French chemist Dr Jean Valnet continued this line of research creating what we now know and accept as the basis of aromatherapy. Today, French doctors take the properties of essential oils as serious medicine whereas those in the United Kingdom see aromatherapy more as a holistic 'alternative' medicine.

While still keeping the technical side of 'Partner Massage and Aroma- therapy' to a minimum, I

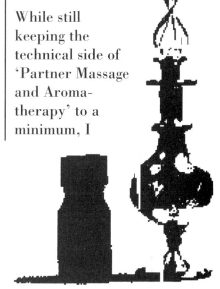

would like to dwell on the practical uses of aromatherapy in our homes and everyday lives.

I see aromatherapy and massage as an on-going thing and not something to be dabbled with once a month or when we sometimes feel like it. Like any exercise, aromatherapy and massage has to be kept going on a regular basis to have any long-term effect. Obviously we can't all afford to go and visit an aromatherapist every week, so most of us tend to visit the former when we are feeling stressed, depressed or plain worn out.

Mind and spirit

I agree that having the occasional massage does wonders for the mind, spirit and body but unfortunately it doesn't provide us with the more long-term effects that it should. I hope that by studying this book you will be in a position to treat yourself and your partner to regular massage without the expense of visiting a professional aromatherapist, masseur or masseuse.

In the following chapter I have listed some of the many essential oils that can be purchased in health shops or by mail order. These are normally readily obtainable. Should you have any problem finding any essential oil that you want, however, it is well worth while writing direct to the makers and blenders of essential oils. You will find this a much cheaper way of eventually obtaining an ample stock of the essential oils of your choice.

Discount

An even cheaper way to obtain pure oils is to get together with a friend or friends and order in bulk from a wholesaler. This way you will probably receive a substantial discount on the oils you purchase. In my early days of massage a few of us got together and managed to build up a

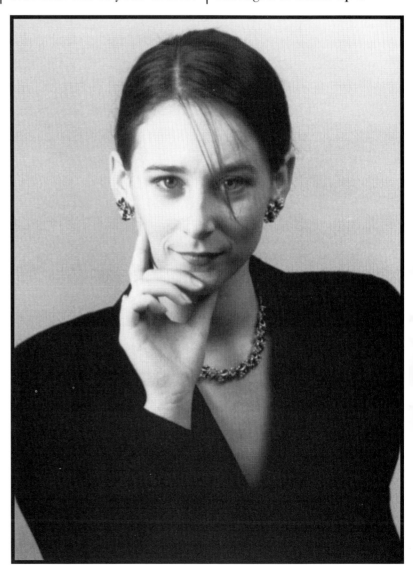

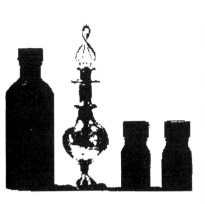

healthy store of oils at a fraction of the price we would normally have paid through local health shops and stores. It is well worth following this up if you are thinking of becoming a serious student of aromatherapy.

Essential oils are highly concentrated and should be used with caution. For massage purposes they are diluted with a vegetable (base) oil, e.g. almond oil. Blend 15–20 drops of the essential oil in 50 ml base oil.

Applications

There are various containers you can use to apply your blend of base oil and your essence/s. When I say 'container' I mean something that you can pour your oil into to make the application of the oil to your partner easy. I have seen various containers.

The most popular seems to be a small liqueur glass, while others prefer an egg cup or small bowl of a similar size. They dip their fingers into the bowl and apply it to their hands.

Physical contact

I have never liked finger-bowl applications, as I either do not get enough oil onto my fingers or it tends to drip off before I have time to apply it to my other hand. This means dipping yet again for more oil.

You may remember that in the section 'massage do's and don'ts' I said it was important not to lose physical contact with your partner during a massage. Because of this, I favour a small pliable plastic container with a nozzle, similar to a miniature washing-up liquid bottle, which allows you to squeeze the contents into your palm.

Containers

If you are able to discover a chemist that sells such

bottles, then you are lucky. I have two such containers and guard them with my life. While I pour oil from this type of container into my right hand I keep my forearm or back of my right wrist against my client's arm, hip, foot, or whatever, so as not to lose contact.

Disorientated

I remember receiving a massage where the masseuse lost contact with me for some period of time. At the time I was drifting in and out of sleep when I suddenly woke, startled and disorientated. I was suddenly on my own. Because of this personal experience I have never lost physical contact with my client since.

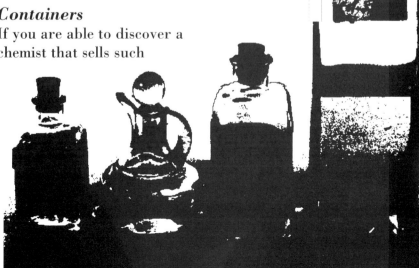

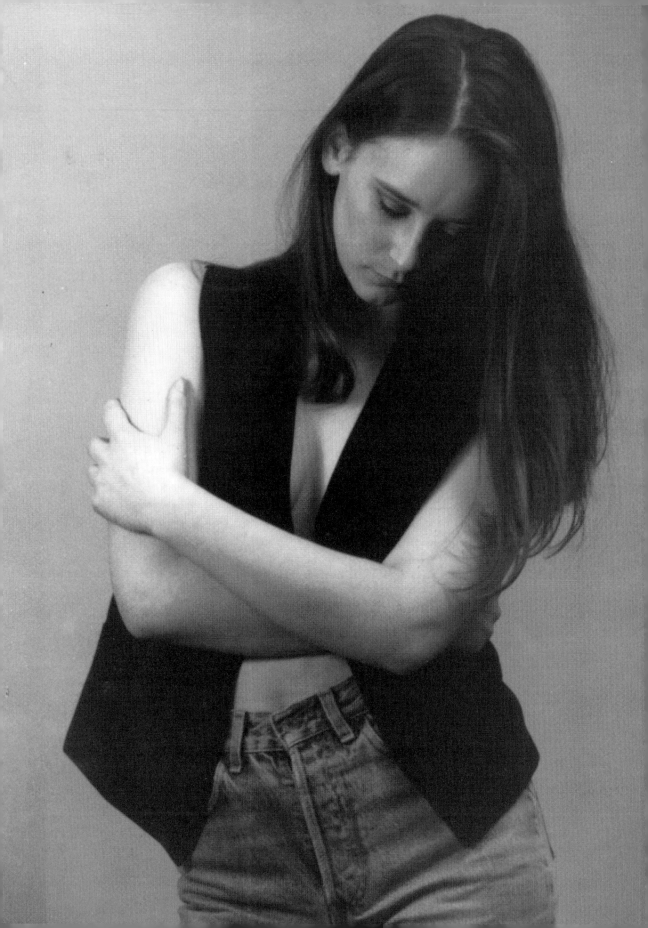

essential oils

The fragrance of essential oils influence the mood, because they have an effect on the areas of the brain concerned with our emotions. Combined with massage, essential oils can be used to treat a wide range of ailments.

Essential oils are very powerful and should be used sensibly. As mentioned in the previous chapter, use only a few drops of essential oil diluted in a Base oil for massage purposes.

Listed below are the most commonly used oils and their possible applications. Please note that some oils can cause skin irritation. There are some precautions which must be taken into account when using the oils. These are indicated in italics under the relevant oil.

Angelica
Angelica archangelica

The oil of angelica is extracted from the roots and seeds. It helps eliminate toxins and excess body fluids, relieves *gout* and *arthritis*, fevers, colds, indigestion, PMT and menopause problems, and also stress-related symptoms such as migraine, headache and mental fatigue. Try it also as a skin tonic.
Not to be used by diabetics.

Basil, French
Ocimum basilicum

Has a calming yet uplifting effect and is excellent for those who simply feel worn out and stressed. Basil will also help with sinus congestion, fainting, insomnia, poor memory, the ability to concentrate, mental stimulation and anxiety.
May irritate sensitive skin.

Bay, West Indian
Pimenta racemosa

Helps to stimulate the circulation, and has long been used as a hair tonic as it stimulates the blood vessels of the hair follicles. Add a few drops to your shampoo when washing your hair. This oil also

helps sprains, rheumatism, colds, flu and insomnia.
Use in moderation.

Benzoin
Styrax benzoin

An antiseptic oil of particular use for urinary infections and skin impurities. It has a warming and relaxing effect. Useful for conditions such as dry skin, blisters and sadness.

Bergamot
Citrus bergamia

Bergamot has an uplifting, sweet and fruity scent and can be used either in base oil or bath water. Depression, shyness, lack of confidence, anxiety, obsession, despondency, negative thoughts, painful digestion, loss of appetite and travel sickness are but a few of its applications.
Phototoxic, so do not apply when about to be exposed to the sun.

Black Pepper
Piper nigrum

As its name suggests, this is a hot essence and can be helpful with colds, aches and pains, influenza, flatulence and rheumatism.

It also stimulates the bowels and aids digestion, eases arthritis and is good after sports activity, sickness, and stomach pains. It is also purported to be of help in relieving tension.
May irritate sensitive skin.

Cajuput
Melaleuca leucodendron

A strong camphoraceous oil, analgesic and antiseptic, it is mainly used for respiratory ailments such as colds, coughs, sore throats, laryngitis and sinus infections. It is also useful for toothache, earache, psoriasis and acne.
May irritate sensitive skin.

Cardamom
Elettaria cardamomum

A warm, spicy aromatic oil that is a good digestive aid. As well as indigestion it helps in the treatment of nausea, diarrhoea, flatulence, colic and confusion.
May irritate sensitive skin.

Carrot
Daucus carota

Helpful in gout, ulcers, flatulence, eczema and psoriasis. It acts as a diuretic.

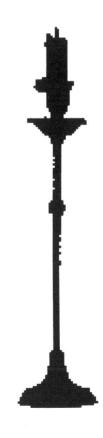

Cedarwood
Cedrus atlantica

Can be used in the treatment of colds, coughs, oily hair and skin, acne, dandruff, arthritis and stress.

Chamomile
Matricaria chamomile

Has many uses and is notably helpful in the treatment of period pains, hot flushes, insomnia, inflammation, stomach cramps, burns, migraine, dermatitis, eczema, skin irritation, psoriasis, nettle rash, swollen joints, gout, frayed nerves, a restless mind, worry and bad temper.

Citronella
Cymbopogon nardus

This oil can be used as an insecticide or deodorant, though it is mainly used as an air freshener. Citronella is related to lemon-grass and has a fresh, sweet, lemony aroma.

Clary-sage
Salvia sclarea

Helpful in strengthening the nervous system and in the treatment of anxiety and depression. This oil can also be used as a sedative and to treat insomnia, negativity, claustrophobia, hyperactivity, mental strain, exhaustion, hostility, sulking and PMT.

Clove
Eugenia caryophyllata

Has a strong, stimulative effect on the mind and body and is reported to have aphrodisiac properties. Clove has traditionally been used to deaden the pain of toothache. It is also a strong antiseptic, helping to clear up sores, and repels insects. *Use in moderation.*

Coriander
Coriandrum sativum

Helpful in the treatment of indigestion, influenza, fatigue, rheumatism, flatulence and nervousness. It is an analgesic, aids the memory and is good for lack of appetite. Coriander is said to be an aphrodisiac. *Stupefying in large quantities, use in moderation.*

Cypress
Cypressus sempervirens

Cypress is purported to have a host of applications. For example, it is said to be helpful in the treatment of varicose veins, haemorr-hoids, whooping cough, nervous tension, wounds, nose bleeds, cellulite, chesti-ness, frequent urination, heavy periods, menopausal problems, bed-wetting, sweaty feet, and even jealousy.

Dill
Anethum graveolens

Not a commonly used oil but it is said to be helpful in the treatment of flatulence, indigestion, constipation, gastric upsets, nervousness and headaches. It is specially useful for children's tummy problems.

Eucalyptus
Eucalyptus globulus

A strong camphoraceous oil that is warming and antiseptic. It is useful as a steam inhalant for heavy colds and nasal congestion, catarrh, bronchitis, sinusitis or asthma. Use it also for wounds and burns, and as a repellent for mosquitoes and gnats. A small drop on a tissue or pillow when you sleep at night will help to relieve a blocked up nose and congested chest.

Eucalyptus, Lemon
Eucalyptus citriodora

Said to be good for the treatment of dandruff, scabs, sores, candida, fungal infections and asthma.

Frankincense
Boswellia thurifera

This remarkable oil has been around for a very long time and its qualities are said to be of tremendous help in harmonising, healing and rejuvenating the whole system. It restores elasticity to the tissues and helps towards relieving anxiety and tension, fear, panic attacks, paranoia, nightmares, irritability, nervousness, apprehension and claustrophobia. It is also said to aid meditation.

Geranium
Pelargonium graveolens

Decongestant, antiseptic and analgesic, this oil can be used as an antiseptic for the skin (specially helpful in cases of dry eczema). It is very calming, helps in mood swings, and is good for hormone imbalance such as PMT, for menopausal problems and impotence.

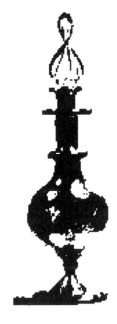

Ginger
Zingiber officinale

A warm and stimulating oil, which is antiseptic and helps combat tonsillitis, colds, flu and sore throats. It is useful too in the treatment of nausea and digestive disorders, such as diarrhoea and bilious attacks. It helps angina, rheumatism and arthritis. A remarkable oil containing excellent properties.

Grapefruit
Citrus paradisi

A detoxifying and astringent oil, grapefruit is helpful in the treatment of obesity, kidney and liver problems, migraine and depression. It is also purported to be useful as an aid in drug withdrawal and for jealousy, envy, despondency, frustration, procrastination and indecisiveness.

Jasmine
Jasminum officinale

An exotic, warm oil that has an uplifting effect. A good relaxant, it is used in the treatment of nervous tension, depression, anxiety, lethargy and menstrual problems. It is also considered as an aphrodisiac, and to be helpful for secretive, sad or shy persons and whenever there is apathy or stress.

Lavender
Lavendula angustifolium (L. officinalis, L. spica)

One of the most commonly used and among the safest essential oils. It is antiseptic, kind to the skin and specially good for the treatment of skin inflammations, wounds, burns, blisters, cuts, sores and bites. Lavender also relieves migraine, nausea, nervous tension, asthma, bacterial infections, acne, boils, rheumatism and arthritis, and cystitis. It appears to boost the immune system. The oil is also very effective in keeping midges, gnats and mosquitoes at bay. Lavender oil is definitely a 'must' for every bathroom cabinet.

Lemon
Citrus limonum

A strongly antiseptic oil, helpful in the treatment of greasy skin, bites and boils and other minor skin conditions, warts, verrucae, cellulite, wrinkles, brittle nails, inflammation of the eyelids, candida, herpes,

migraine, high blood pressure and digestive problems, respiratory tract infections such as colds, bronchitis and sinusitis. Lemon oil can be diluted as a gargle for tonsilitis and inflammation of the gums. This is yet another 'must' for the bathroom cabinet. Lemon can also be used as an insect repellent.
Phototoxic, so do not use when about to sunbathe.

Lemon-grass
Cymbopogon citratus

An excellent pick-me-up, anti-bacterial, and good in the treatment of acne and other skin problems, respiratory problems, sore throats, fevers, headaches and nervous exhaustion. It is excellent, too, as an insect-repellant.

Lime
Citrus aurantifolia

For the treatment of oily skin, fevers, anorexia, depression and anxiety.
The oil made with the peel is Phototoxic.

Mandarin
Citrus nobilis

Mandarin has a delicate and gentle aroma. It has a stimulating effect on the stomach and liver and a calming effect on the intestines. It is therefore good in cases of digestive disorders. Use it for anxiety and insomnia as well.

Marjoram
Origanum marjorana

Marjoram is excellent for uplifting the spirits and for a feeling of general well-being. An analgesic, it soothes aching muscles and is good for sprains, bruises, intestinal cramps, menstrual problems, insomnia, bronchitis and asthma.

Melissa
Melissa officinalis

Beneficial and soothing to the mind and body. Helps to lower high blood pressure and is used as a sedative, for nervousness, palpitations and stress.It can also be used to treat allergies, bacterial and fungal infections, eczema and heavy periods.
Can irritate sensitive skin.

Myrrh
Commiphora myrrha

Helpful in the treatment of gums and for mouth ulcers.

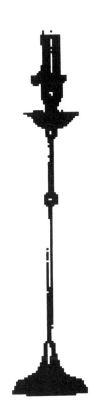

It can also be used to treat respiratory infections (such as colds and sore throats) and catarrh, fungal infections, candida and dermatitis. This oil is rejuvenating to the whole system.

Neroli
Citrus aurantium

Derived from orange blossom, neroli oil is a mild sedative and antidepressant. It can be recommended for the treatment of emotional problems or when there is any emotional shock. Neroli should be considered in cases of hysteria, anxiety, palpitations, insomnia, dermatitis, dry skin, disorientation, mental strain, overwork and menopausal problems.

Orange
Citrus aurantium

Orange oil, which is expressed from the peel of the fruit, has very similar properties to neroli. It is antiseptic, antidepressant, antispasmodic and a mild sedative, particularly good in the treatment of nervous conditions, lack of energy or for constipation.
Phototoxic so do not use before exposure to the sun.

Patchouli
Pogostemon patchouli

Anti-inflammatory and antiseptic, this oil is useful in skin care and the treatment of conditions such as dandruff, acne and eczema.

Peppermint
Mentha piperata

Commonly used for the treatment of digestive disorders. Its warming properties can be helpful at the start of a cold. Try it also for travel sickness, nausea, flatulence, headaches, migraine, liver problems, toothache, sunburn, bilious attacks, and as a mental stimulant. It can be used as a foot-bath for tired and aching feet, and is also an effective mosquito repellent.
Use in moderation.

Pine
Pinus sylvestris

Excellent for the treatment of chest infections. Inhalations of pine help to relieve the misery of colds, catarrh and sore throats (the oil is an antiseptic). Pine is also good for the treatment of muscular aches and pains, lumbago, cystitis and kidney problems, PMT, sweaty feet and lice. *Avoid using on allergic skin conditions.*

Rose
Rosa damascena

A rather expensive oil but of great benefit in helping to regulate the menstrual cycle and as a tonic for the whole system. Rose helps emotionally by acting as an antidepressant. The oil is also good for circulatory problems, loss of appetite, hay fever, wrinkles, broken capillaries, nervous eczema and psoriasis.

Sandalwood
Santalum album

A powerful antiseptic in the treatment of cystitis, skin complaints (such as acne), nausea, and fungal and bacterial infections. Sandal-wood is useful for menstrual problems and impotence. It is a fine relaxant, helpful in the practice of meditation and also regarded as an aphrodisiac.

Tea-tree
Melaleuca alternifolia

A strong antiseptic invaluable in combating bacterial, viral and fungal infections. It is of particular benefit in the treatment of colds and cold sores, warts, verrucae, burns, candida, athlete's foot, impetigo, vaginitis, and ear, nose and throat infections. Tea-tree can also be used as a gargle for sufferers of halitosis.

Violet
Viola odorata

Not a commonly used essence but valuable as a liver decongestant and for relieving fibrositis, kidney problems, and skin conditions such as acne and eczema.

Ylang-ylang
Cananga odorata

Ylang-ylang can be used in the treatment of numerous ailments and conditions, such as emotional shock, fear (it regulates rapid breathing), high blood pressure, insomnia, impotence and frigidity (this oil is said to be an

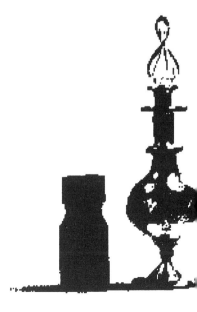

aphrodisiac). It can also be used as a sedative, and general tonic. If you ever suffer from panic attacks, nervousness, stress, impatience or anger, a few drops of this oil on your pillow or handkerchief will help to relieve these symptoms.

Finally, I'd like to mention two widely used but very much underestimated herb plants that have been utilised for many thousands of years   garlic and onion. Both these bulbs are old friends of our Mediterranean cousins who for many centuries have used them not only for culinary purposes but for their tremendous cleansing effect on the blood and lymphatic systems. As most people find the odour of garlic and onion pretty powerful the oils are generally taken internally in capsule form.

Garlic
Allium sativum

Garlic is a plant whose healing properties have been known since ancient times. The Egyptians saw garlic as a divine herb. The pyramid workers received a clove of garlic each day because of its antiseptic and health-boosting properties.

The Greeks and Romans saw this simple herb as an all-round ailment cure.

Garlic can be found growing wild in Spain, Egypt, Sicily and Algeria. Though mainly used in cooking, the following is a list of its unusual remedial properties.

Tonic (digestive), general stimulant, circulatory stimulant, slows down the pulse, antispasmodic, glandular restorative, antisclerotic (blood thinning), diuretic, anti-gout, anti-arthritic, aperitif, stomachic, detoxifier, vermifuge, febrifuge, a cancer preventative, decongestant, antiseptic.

Garlic is specially helpful in cases of catarrh, sinusitis, bronchitis, colds, high blood pressure, heart disease, acne, worms, scabies, gastro-intestinal infections.

Onion
Allium cepa

The common onion is another amazing bulbous plant that can be found growing throughout the world. As with garlic, this herb has been around for many centuries and has tremendous healing properties. The following is a list of some of these:

General stimulant, digestive stimulant, diuretic,

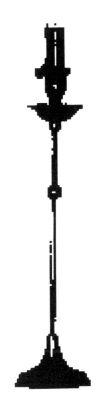

antirheumatic, antiseptic, anti-infection, antibiotic, antithrombosis, vermifuge, mild hypnotic, curative for the skin and hair, decongestant, reputed aphrodisiac.

Onion is recommended for sinusitis, colds, abscesses, haemorrhoids, chilblains and chapped skin, migraine, cerebral congestion, toothache, verrucae, warts, alopecia, freckles, ulcers and burns.

At this point I would like to quote Dr Jean Valnet's passage in his translated book *The Practice of Aromatherapy* (C.W. Daniel) where he states on page 198:

'… may I remind the reader that, like any form of treatment, Aromatherapy does not claim to be effective, by itself, for every ailment, nor for every patient, nor in every circumstance. It must often be used in conjunction with other medications.'

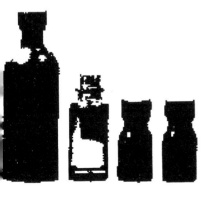

joss 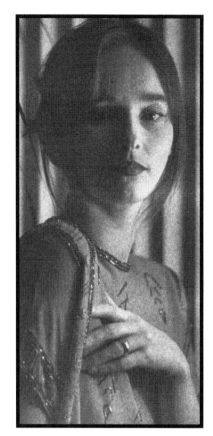15
sticks
and
fragrances

I f we wander down any market place today we are more than likely to come across a stall or small shop committed to selling nothing but 'sensual delicacies'. As there doesn't seem to be a collective name for these shops we could call them a 'health delicatessen'. In these shops we find an array of products to brighten and give pleasant aromas to our homes and bodies.

Pot pourri

It is fun to browse slowly through these shops inhaling the numerous scents that waft from the many pot-pourri, perfumed candles, soaps, dried flowers and joss sticks. I usually come out feeling quite heady from the strength of these aromas.

I am a great believer in burning joss sticks in the home. The pleasant aroma lingers long after the incense has burnt itself out. Burning incense helps remove smells that come from cooking, smoking and the general stuffiness that pervades most homes. With today's traffic pollution it is not always a good idea to leave our windows open for any length of time.

Healthier air

Where I live it is more healthy to keep the windows closed in the day and open at night when the traffic has died down. I have found that any physical exercises that I might care to do are better done with the windows closed. The air in our homes is more often than not far cleaner than that affected by what is going on outside.

So burning incense in the home can bring a strong uplift to the spirits of the occupants. The many aromas given off by incense can produce many different feelings, moods and emotions. When buying incense it is a good idea to read the labels to discover what each aroma's effect has on us. For instance, my favourite is sandalwood. This aroma produces a pleasant mood for me and is good for inducing a meditative mind for writing.

Here is a short list of incenses that, if pure enough, can help relieve the

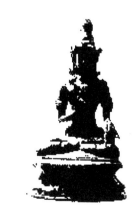

following conditions on the mind and body when burnt. Because there are some differences of opinion about which fragrance does what to whom, I feel we should follow our own instincts regardless of what the many different labels say. If you like the aroma, enjoy it. If you find it sickly or too sweet then don't use it. It's a matter of personal taste and knowing what you like and don't like.

Basil, French
opening

Poor concentration, tired-ness, exhaustion, fatigue, weariness, sluggishness, irritability, lack of attention, poor memory, listlessness, low mental stimulation and lack of self-discipline.

Bergamot
uplifting

Anxiety, remorse, no confidence, depression, despair, negativity, 'the day after the night before' feeling, obsession, feeling frightened and shy, stressed.

Benzoin
soothing

Loneliness, feeling friendless and/or rejected, sadness.

Cajuput
focusing

Compulsiveness, obsession, cynicism, disorientation, poor memory, procrastination, lack of clarity.

Cardamon
expansion

Confusion, selfishness, greed, negativity, bewilderment, clutter.

Cedarwood
composing

Stress, scattered thinking, fragmented mind, anxiety, strain.

Chamomile
soothing

Impulsiveness, overactive or restless mind, impetuousness, tantrums, capriciousness, worry.

Clary-sage
euphoria

Claustrophobia, compulsiveness, depression, bad dreams, hostility, hyperactivity, insomnia, listlessness, negative thoughts, obsession, over-analytical, overwork, mental strain, nervous exhaustion, restlessness with exhaustion, stress, sulking.

Cypress
astringent

Jealousy, sluggishness, talkativeness, envy, possessiveness, resentment, covetousness.

Frankincense
rejuvenating

Apprehension, claustrophobia, timidity, fear, worry, foreboding, dread, insecurity, irritability, nervousness, nightmares, panic attacks, paranoia, self-criticism, instability, lack of discipline or perseverance.

Geranium
harmonious

Attachment, mood swings, rigidity, discord.

Ginger
digestion

Inhibition, lack of self-acceptance or confidence.

Grapefruit
releasing

Bitterness, lack of clarity, confusion, despondency, envy, frustration, indecisiveness, jealousy, procrastination, fear stemming from the past.

Jasmine
aphrodisiac

Apathy, inattention, indifference, inhibited emotional expression, fear of the future, frigidity, jealousy, nit-picking, rigidity, sadness, secretiveness, shyness, stress.

Juniper
toxin dispersal

Lethargy, apathy, indifference.

Lavender
immune system stimulant

Fear, alarm, terror, stage-fright, hysteria, hyperactivity, impatience, insomnia, insecurity, inability to relax, irrationality, irritability, mood swings, negative thoughts, worry about the future, overwork, paranoia, restlessness, overactive

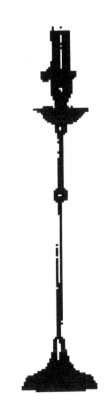

mind, apprehension, panic
attacks, trepidation,
horror.

Lemon
refreshing

Selfishness, sluggishness,
languor, lethargy,
droopiness, listlessness.

Lemon-grass
strengthening

Boredom, lack of interest,
overwork, nervous
exhaustion, sulkiness,
languor.

Marjoram
relaxant

Hostility, hyperactivity,
irrational thoughts,
overwork, mental strain,
tension, antagonism,
unfriendliness.

Melissa
sedation

Shock, worry, distress,
fretfulness, being upset or
withdrawn.

Neroli
relief from stress

Bereavement,
disorientation, fright,

hysteria, mental strain,
overwork, alarm, restlessness, exhaustion, shock,
being upset or distressed.

Orange
radiance

Selfishness, egotism,
stubbornness, avarice,
greed, self-indulgence.

Patchouli
pervasive

Apprehension, anxiety,
dread, fear, foreboding,
lack of clarity.

Peppermint
cooling, stimulating

Forgetfulness, poor memory
or concentration, affliction
from noise.

Rose
cleansing

Attachment, bereavement,
grief, fear, nervousness,
worry, anguish, mourning,
sorrow, regret, sadness,
self-centredness, terror.

Rosewood
freshening

Apprehension, day-
dreaming, grumpiness,

fear, dread, foreboding,
anxiety, instability.

Sandalwood
*mental and psychic
stimulant*

Cynicism, recurrent
nightmares, dread, fear of
failure, insecurity,
irritability, listlessness,
nervousness, insecurity,
self-centredness,
insensitivity, lack of
perseverance.

Ylang Ylang
relaxing

Depression, insomnia,
nervous tension,
frustration. Aphrodisiac.

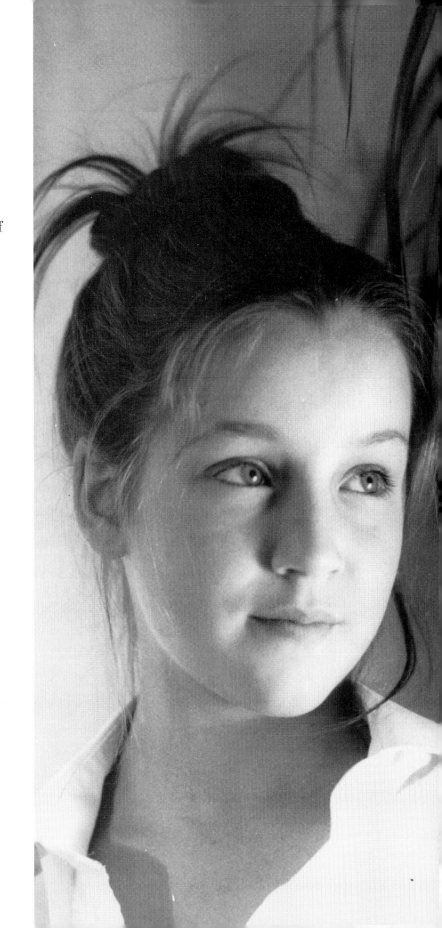

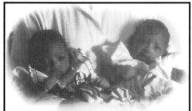

baby talk

Aromatherapy and massage go hand in hand when it comes to pregnancy and childbirth. However, like most things in life, there are dangers and pitfalls to be considered. Essential oils can be powerful friends if used carefully and wisely.

Aromatherapy in relation to childbirth is a subject that requires careful reading and understanding to get the best for you and your baby.

Sensitivity

Within the space of this book I can only touch upon the subject of pregnancy and childbirth, though maybe just enough to encourage you to take the time and energy to follow up with the reading matter of your choice.

Like the child inside, the mother-to-be is unusually sensitive to external influences and stimulants. During pregnancy the mother's body undergoes many changes so as to accommodate the new arrival. Bearing in mind the whole range of oils that have been mentioned in this book, I would now like to add a list of essences that should be avoided during pregnancy. In my research it seems that some aromatherapists differ in their opinion of what is good or bad for the mother and baby to be.

Avoid

Owing to their toxic nature the oils asterisked on the following list are generally accepted as ones to be completely avoided, especially during pregnancy.

Aniseed

Armoise

Arnica*

Basil

Camphor, brown and yellow,

Caraway

Chamomile

Clary sage

Cinnamon bark

Clove

Cedarwood

Fennel

Hyssop

Juniper

Marjoram

Mugwort

Myrrh

Nutmeg

Origanum

Parsley

Peppermint

Pennyroyal*

Rose

Rosemary

Sage

Savory

Tansy*

Tarragon

Thuja*

Thyme

Wintergreen*

Consultation with a qualified aromatherapist would be wise before using any of the oils in the above list during pregnancy.

Massage in pregnancy is particularly helpful throughout the later stages. Massage helps to calm and relieve some of the stress and discomfort felt in the spine caused by the increase of weight in the uterus. The benefits of massage can also be felt throughout labour. Pain is eased and your newborn profits greatly too.

Stretch marks
Due to the stretching of the skin during pregnancy the mother often suffers from permanent stretch marks. Massage the stomach twice a day with a mixture of 20 drops of lavender in a 50 ml base oil of wheatgerm or almond. This routine should considerably reduce these marks.

Morning sickness
The use of lavender can be of help in relieving the morning sickness that most pregnant mothers experience in the early weeks. A few drops of lavender oil added to your bath water or dabbed on your night clothes or pillow will not only help reduce the nausea but also the anxiety that often comes with pregnancy.

If you find you are oversensitive to smells at this time, an essence burner (see page 14) with a few drops of lavender added will help dispel most offending odours. Lavender is one of those precious oils that can be of help towards dispelling a multitude of ailments.

Baby massage
To gently massage your newborn can be of tremendous psychological help and support to him or her in later years. I have already said in this book that most of us lack the touch that we should have experienced when we were young. Most people are disturbed when touched or caressed in later life. This is due to the absence of hugs and caresses in our early years. We have grown up insulated from love and caring. We don't trust.

Parents who love their children should take the time to show their feelings through physical contact with their offspring throughout their child's formative years. Only this tactile contact will sustain the caring and love that is so desperately missing in society today.

Begin massaging and stroking your child in the way that only a mother or father can from the day that he or she is born. There is no need for oils your touch will be enough.

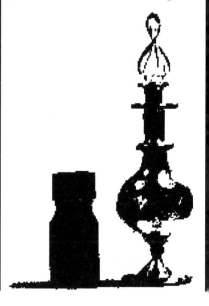

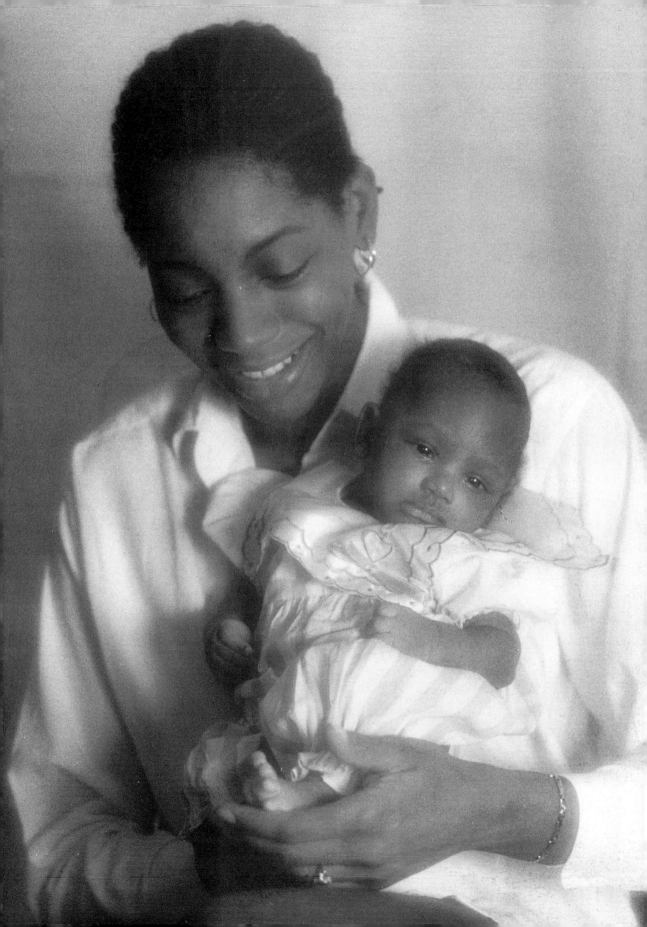

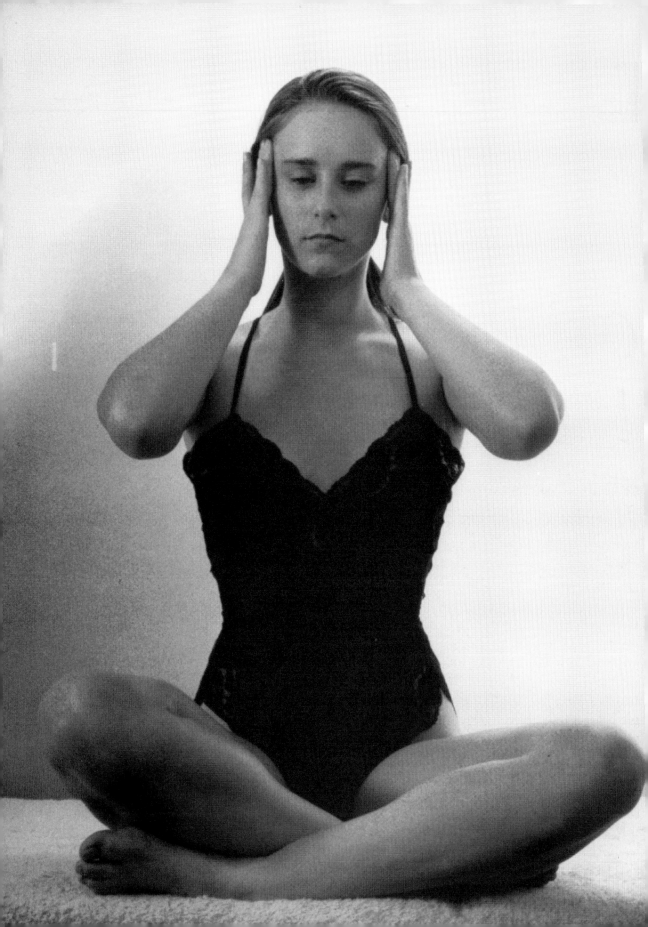

other techniques

Reflexology

Reflexology dates back to ancient China, and has an effect on our body through stimulating certain points on the sole of the foot that correspond to the body's organs and glands. It therefore works on the whole body. This therapy would be termed as complementary medicine and falls under the heading of holistic healing.

Our feet are intended to take us from place to place, but in this day and age the various forms of transport offered to us hardly allow our feet to get the exercise that they were originally intended to receive. What with fashionable shoes that crimp our feet, together with concrete roads and pavements, our feet are insulated from the ground we walk upon. Our feet hardly touch the ground. A good experiment to find out how sensitive our feet are would be to stroll across a pebbled beach or path. I

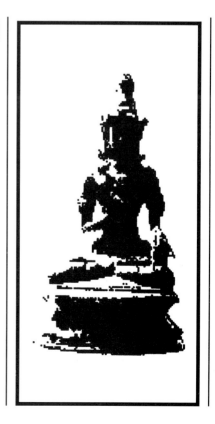

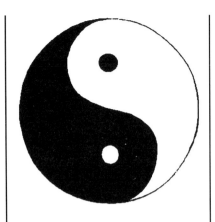

for one hobble painfully from one foot to the other while children never seem to notice any discomfort whatsoever. Their feet are supple and their bodies basically in harmony, while us shoe-conscious oldies are usually way out of balance. So, reflexology helps towards regaining the bodily balance and harmony that was once ours.

Reflexology, like acupuncture, works on our reflex zones or meridians. By exerting pressure on specific points, blockages in our energy pathways are able to clear themselves.

This therapy assists the body to heal itself. The sole of the foot is a reflection of our whole body and contains zones representing all our organs and bodily functions.

Depth

Like aromatherapy, reflexology is a subject that has tremendous depth in its own right and couldn't possibly be explained in the short section allowed for in this book. However, I will endeavour to cover the basics so that you can couple this with body massage and include it in the treatment of your partner. There is nothing more pleasant and relaxing than receiving a good foot massage before a full body massage. Try it and see.

Stress

Not surprisingly stress is one of the main culprits underlying disease of the mind and body. All holistic therapies are based on this assumption. The

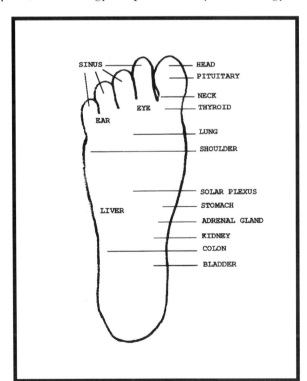

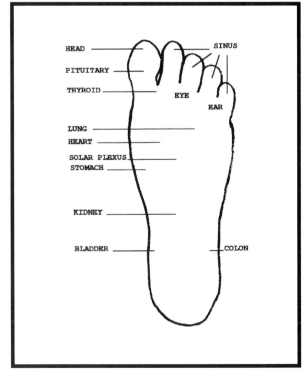

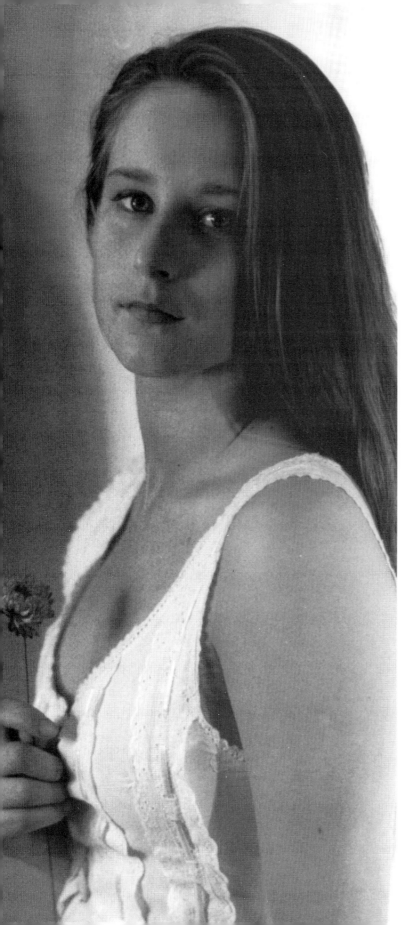

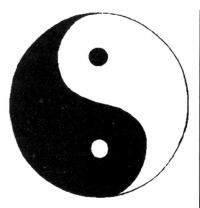

eradication of the results and reasons for stress is the aim. By following the diagram of the main areas of the foot you can give attention to your partner's feet either before or during your body massage.

It is far better either to massage the foot with talcum powder or just dry hands than to apply a base oil, which would create a slippery surface and inhibit the friction required.

Warmth

With your partner lying on his or her back on the bed or floor, begin by gently rubbing the whole foot with both hands to generate warmth in it and bring about relaxation.

Stroking

Next apply gentle but firm pressure to the sole of the foot either by making small circles or by stroking

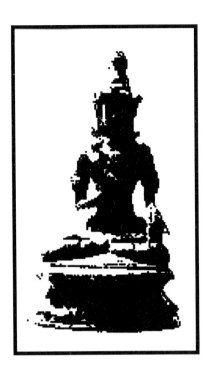

movements with your thumbs on the areas depicted in the diagram, from toe to heel on each foot.

Shiatsu

Shiatsu (finger pressure) is a Japanese therapy closely related to acupuncture. Unlike other forms of massage, clients keep their clothes on and the treatment is performed either on the floor or on a low couch or table.

Like acupuncture, shiatsu is based on the idea that the life energy, called chi, flows through the body in what are called meridians. These meridians are linked to the body's major organs.

It is thought that if the energy is blocked the linked organ is not able to function properly and the person becomes sick or ill. The treatment is vigorous in so far that the therapist presses on the selected channels, using either their knee, elbows or feet.

Swedish Massage

Swedish massage is different from other forms of massage. It involves more vigorous movements such as cupping, pummelling and hacking, and goes slightly deeper. The style is invigorating as opposed to a more flowing action.

Toxins

For people who have unknowingly built up toxins in their body, Swedish massage helps drain the lymphatic system and helps to improve circulation.

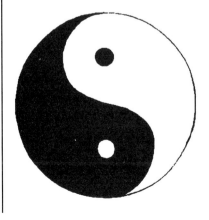

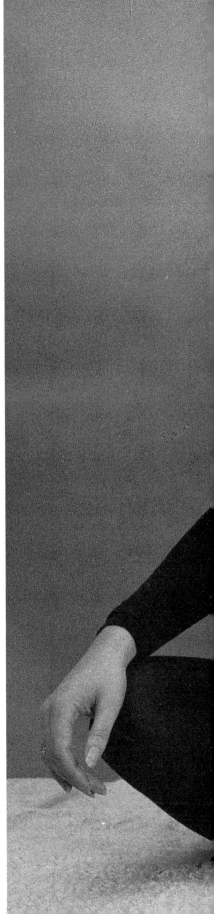

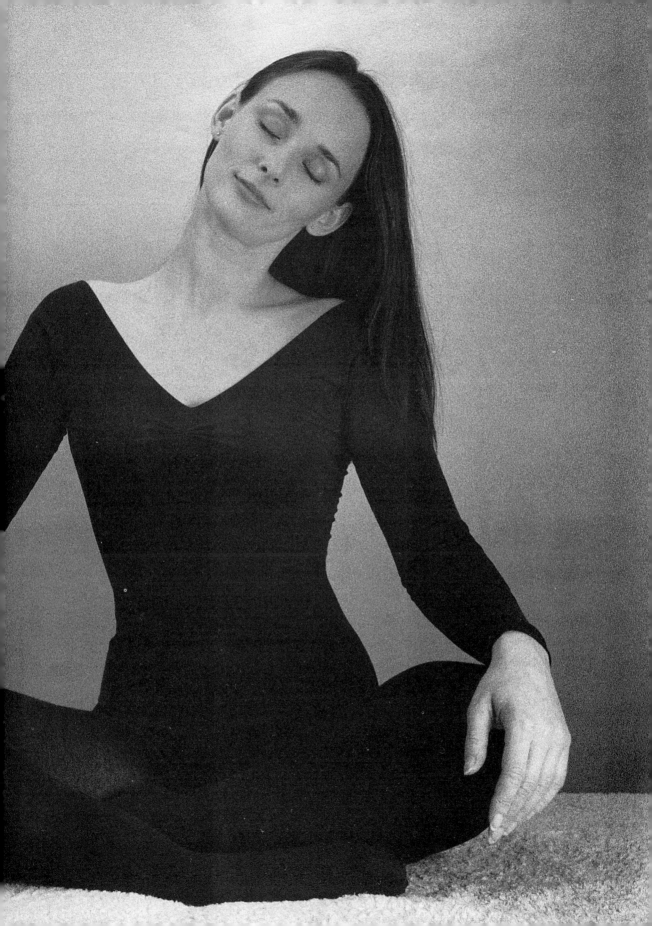

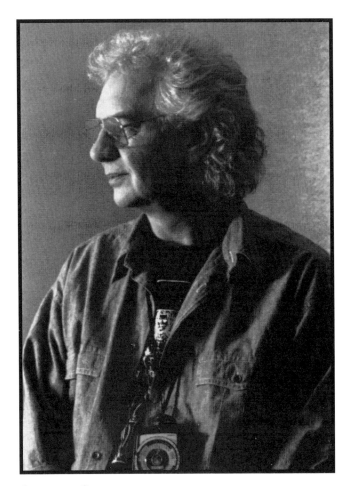

brian green